SMALL ANIMAL OPHTHALMOLOGY:
A Problem – Oriented Approach

ROBERT L. PEIFFER, JR., DVM, PhD, ACVO

Associate Professor and Director of
Laboratories, Department of Ophthalmology,
School of Medicine, The University of North
Carolina at Chapel Hill, Chapel Hill

with five contributors

A SAUNDERS VETERINARY QUICK REFERENCE HANDBOOK

W. B. SAUNDERS COMPANY
Harcourt Brace Jovanovich, Inc.
Philadelphia, London, Toronto, Montreal, Sydney, Tokyo

W. B. SAUNDERS COMPANY

Harcourt Brace Jovanovich, Inc.

The Curtis Center
Washington Square West
Philadelphia, PA 19106

Library of Congress Cataloging-in-Publication Data

Small animal ophthalmology : a problem-oriented approach / [compiled
   by] Robert L. Peiffer, Jr.
      p.   cm.
   ISBN 0-7216-1461-2
   1. Dogs—Diseases. 2. Cats—Diseases. 3. Veterinary
ophthalmology.   I. Peiffer, Robert L.
SF992.E92S63 1989
636.7'08977—dc19   88-29851
                                                                   CIP

SMALL ANIMAL OPHTHALMOLOGY:
   A Problem-Oriented Approach   ISBN   0-7216-1461-2

Last digit is the print number: 9   8   7   6   5   4   3

SAUNDERS VETERINARY QUICK REFERENCE HANDBOOKS

Published

Reedy and Miller: Allergic Skin Diseases of the Dog and Cat

Forthcoming

Tams: Small Animal Gastroenterology

Brobst, Parry and Foreyt: Veterinary Laboratory Tests

Loar, Rosenthal and Susaneck: Small Animal Clinical Oncology

Crowe, Kovacic and Kirby: Veterinary Emergency and Trauma Care

Dedicated

to

our patients

Contributors

CYNTHIA S. COOK, D.V.M, PH.D.

Assistant Research Anatomist, Department of Growth and Development, University of California at San Francisco; Staff Ophthalmologist, Animal Eye Clinic, Menlo Park, California

Clinical Basic Science; Orbital or Ocular Pain

BEVERLEY COTTRELL, M.A.VET., M.B., CERT. V. OPHTHAL., M.R.C.V.S.

Comparative Ophthalmology Unit, Animal Health Trust, Newmarket, Suffolk, England

Abnormal Appearance

DENNIS V. HACKER, D.V.M., DIPLOMATE, A.C.V.O.

Assistant Clinical Professor, V.M.T.H., University of California at Davis

Diagnostics; Therapeutics

ARNOLD LEON, B.V.M.&S., CERT. V. OPHTHAL., M.R.C.V.S.

Research Assistant, Comparative Ophthalmology Unit, Animal Health Trust, Newmarket, Suffolk, England

Visual Impairment

ROBERT L. PEIFFER, JR., D.V.M., PH.D., DIPLOMATE, A.C.V.O.

Professor, Departments of Ophthalmology and Pathology, School of Medicine, University of North Carolina at Chapel Hill

Abnormal Appearance; Ocular Discharge

SIMON M. PETERSEN-JONES, B.VET.MED., D.V.OPHTHAL., M.R.C.V.S.

Lectures in Ophthalmology, University of Edinburgh

Ocular Discharge

Acknowledgments

Confucius stated that a man must do three things to achieve immortality: plant a tree, have a son, and write a book. Having experienced all, I can state that the latter is probably the most challenging! We are indebted to all who made this venture possible; myself to my contributors, and all of us to those who lent support in terms of time, encouragement, logistics, and information. This includes our families, secretaries, colleagues, and mentors. Special thanks to Ms. Janet Yarbrough for her work in manuscript preparation and to David Eifrig, Chairman of Ophthalmology at UNC, who has always had the enlightened perspective of "one medicine" that has allowed me to pursue my comparative interests within the framework of a medical school department. Not least, the patience, support, and expertise of Darlene Pedersen, editor, and W.B. Saunders Company have been most instrumental in bringing our creation to fruition.

Time is the ultimate judge of all endeavors. May our arbors flourish, our children prosper, and our readers find value in this text.

Preface

Ophthalmology has blossomed and matured as a recognized, valued specialty of veterinary medicine and surgery; ophthalmic exposure is generally emphasized in the professional curriculum; the competency and sophistication of the general practitioner is continually improving; and several excellent contemporary comprehensive textbooks are available on the subject.

Then why this text? We have recognized a need by the general practitioner for an informative source that he or she can turn to as a guide to the management of a particular problem. Appropriate management implies two inseparable principles—accurate diagnosis and adequate therapy. We have attempted to address each with equal emphasis. We perceive a need by the student for a text that condenses a large amount of information into a "friendly" manual that emphasizes problem solving rather than memorization and that provides more usable information than lecture notes without the depth of a reference text. We hope this manual meets these needs.

Why these authors? The profession and the specialty are evolving and changing. Although I am somewhat reluctant to classify myself as "mature" as a clinical ophthalmologist, I cannot help but be impressed by the energy, enthusiasm, and ideas of a younger generation of amazingly well-trained ophthalmologists. All of the contributors fit this mold, and I hope that they and their colleagues who follow will continue to probingly question the established as well as addressing unsolved problems. Experience is almost always tainted by dogmatism, which in turn can cloud truth; I have encouraged Drs. Cook, Leon, Cottrell, and Petersen-Jones to express their ideas and philosophies without unwarranted respect for sacred cows. The product is exciting.

We have attempted not to reproduce a comprehensive text but to produce a clinical manual; references are not included. As conditions may present with more than one presenting sign, there is some repetition; conditions are discussed in detail under their most obvious or significant sign. We have discussed in detail only those surgical procedures that are likely to be routinely performed by the practitioner, and details of these procedures are described with their pictorial presentation rather than in the text. Emphasis is placed on techniques that have proven to be most valuable and effective for the authors, and readers should recognize that there may indeed by quite acceptable alternative approaches to clinical problems. We do hope that this handbook will prove a ready and valuable reference to the general practitioner presented with a challenging ophthalmic case and when viewed in its entirety will provide a practical overall approach to small animal ophthalmology.

ROBERT L. PEIFFER, JR.
Chapel Hill, N.C.

Contents

5

Abnormal Appearance

Beverley Cottrell and Robert L. Peiffer, Jr.

6

Orbital or Ocular Pain **195**

Cynthia S. Cook

7

Ocular Discharge **215**

Simon M. Petersen-Jones and Robert L. Peiffer, Jr.

1 | Clinical Basic Science

Cynthia S. Cook

OCULAR EMBRYOLOGY

The ocular primordia appear during the first weeks of gestation as bilateral evaginations of the neural ectoderm of the forebrain. These optic sulci gradually enlarge and approach the surface ectoderm as optic vesicles connected to the forebrain by the optic stalks. Thickening of the overlying surface ectoderm to form the lens placode occurs as a result of inductive influences by the optic vesicle. Invagination of the lens placode occurs concurrently with that of the optic vesicle to form a hollow lens vesicle within a bilayered optic cup, the inner layer of which will form the stratified layers of the neural retina and the inner epithelial layer of the iris and ciliary body; the outer layer becomes the cuboidal, monolayered retinal pigment epithelium, the outer epithelial layer of the iris and ciliary body, and the pupillary sphincter and dilator muscles.

Invagination to form the optic cup occurs eccentrically, with formation of a slitlike opening called the *optic (choroid) fissure* located inferiorly. The vascular supply to the embryonic eye, the hyaloid artery (primary vitreous), enters the optic cup through this opening and branches extensively around the lens to form the tunica vasculosa lentis. Embryonic remnants of this vascular structure may persist as a persistent hyperplastic primary vitreous (PHPV) and/or persistent tunica vasculosa lentis (PTVL). Failure of the optic fissure to close normally may result in congenital defects anteriorly (iridial coloboma) or posteriorly (chorioretinal or optic nerve coloboma). Microphthalmos may occur as a result of deficiencies in the early formation of the optic sulcus or vesicle or from incomplete closure of the optic fissure with failure to establish early intraocular pressure.

The posterior lens epithelial cells elongate, forming primary lens fibers that obliterate the space within the lens vesicle. Secondary lens fibers are formed by elongation of cells at the equator (lens bow); these fibers pass circumferentially around the embryonal lens nucleus.

Thickening of the future neural retina occurs with segregation into inner and outer neuroblastic layers. Cellular proliferation takes place in the outer neuroblastic layer with migration to the inner layer. The ganglion cells are the first to achieve final differentiation, extending axons that form the nerve fiber layer and join as the optic nerve. The horizontal, amacrine, and Müller cells also differentiate in the inner neuroblastic layer. The bipolar cells and photoreceptors develop in the outer neuroblastic layer and form the inner and outer nuclear layers in the adult. Retinal dysplasia may result from disorganized development of the neural retina with formation of folds and rosettes.

Following detachment of the lens vesicle from the surface ectoderm, development of the anterior chamber structures progresses. A specialized population of the neural ectoderm called *neural crest cells* migrates under the surface ectoderm to form the corneal endothelium which secretes its basement membrane, Descemet's membrane. Additional neural crest cells form the corneal stroma between the surface epithelium and endothelium. The anterior iris stroma also develops from neural crest cells migrating onto the anterior surface of the optic cup. Neural crest cells also form the outer two coats of the posterior globe, the choroid (including the tapetum) and sclera.

OCULAR ANATOMY, PHYSIOLOGY, AND BIOCHEMISTRY

Orbit

The orbit in the cat and dog is formed by contributions of the frontal, palatine, lacrimal, maxillary, zygomatic, and presphenoid bones. The bony orbit is incomplete superiotemporally, where it is bridged by the dense orbital ligament, spanning between the frontal process of the zygomatic bone and the zygomatic process of the frontal bone. The lacrimal gland lies superiorly, under this orbital ligament. The orbital contents are covered by a connective tissue layer of periorbita, which is continuous at the limbus with Tenon's capsule. Seven extraocular muscles innervated by the third, fourth, and sixth cranial nerves control movement of the globe. There is a variable amount of fat between the periorbita and the bony wall and surrounding the extraocular muscles. The zygomatic salivary gland is located inferiotemporally, deep to the zygomatic arch, and may be a site of infection or mucocele formation.

The wall of the bony orbital wall is thinner medially and may allow extension of infectious or neoplastic processes originating in the nasal cavity or periorbital sinuses. Infectious processes involving the roots of the molar teeth may also extend to involve the orbit.

Space-occupying orbital lesions include both inflammatory and neoplastic etiologies. Due to the incomplete nature of the bony orbit, both inferiorly and superiotemporally, a space-occupying process may become quite advanced before exophthalmos and/or deviation of the globe is noted. Diagnosis and management of such conditions are discussed in subsequent chapters.

Eyelids

The eyelids form the initial barrier to mechanical damage to the eye. They also serve to distribute the tear film and, through the meibomian glands, provide an oily secretion to slow tear evaporation. The eyelids consist of:

1. An outer layer of thin, pliable skin
2. A small amount of loose connective tissue containing modified sweat glands and the circumferential fibers of the orbicularis oculi muscle (innervated by branches of the facial nerve)
3. The more rigid fibrous connective tissue of the tarsal plate
4. The radial fibers of the levator palpebrae superioris (innervated by the oculomotor nerve) and Müller's (sympathetic innervation via branches of the oculomotor nerve) muscles
5. The palpebral conjunctiva containing goblet cells.

Cilia are found on the margin of the upper lid; posterior to these follicles are the openings of the sebaceous (meibomian) glands (Figures 1-1 and 1-2). Dysplasia or metaplasia of these glands results in formation of aberrant hair follicles (distichia), which may contact the cornea and result in epiphora and, rarely, keratitis.

Surgical manipulations of the eyelids require delicate handling to minimize swelling and careful apposition of surgical or traumatic wound margins. Particular attention should be paid to maintenance of a smooth eyelid margin. Closure of full-thickness defects should utilize a two-layer pattern; the tarsal plate has the greatest strength and should be included in the subcutaneous layer.

Lacrimal System

The precorneal tear film consists of three distinct layers: (1) a mucous layer located closest to the cornea and produced by the conjunctival goblet cells, (2) a thick aqueous layer, and (3) an outer oily layer produced by the meibomian glands of the eyelids. The aqueous portion of the tear film is the combined product of the orbital lacrimal gland and a gland located at the

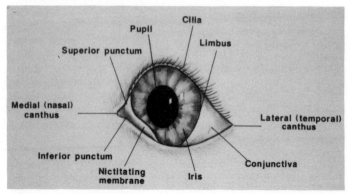

FIGURE 1-1. External appearance of the canine eye (with the exception of the pupillary shape, the feline is identical) depicting the adnexal structures.

base of the third eyelid. The major lacrimal gland is located in the superiotemporal area of the orbit beneath the orbital ligament and supraorbital process of the frontal bone; its secretions appear through numerous small ducts in the superior fornix. The tears are distributed over the surface of the cornea through the action of the eyelids and exit through the nasolacrimal puncta. These two openings are located nasally, superior and inferior to the medial canthus, just inside the eyelid margin (Figure 1-1). The puncta open into two canaliculi joining to form the nasolacrimal duct, which passes through a bony canal in the maxilla to open ventrolaterally in the nasal cavity.

Conjunctiva and Third Eyelid

The *conjunctiva* is a mucous membrane that covers the globe between the fornix and the cornea, the third eyelid, and the inner surface of the eyelids (Figure 1-2). Over the surface of the globe, the conjunctiva blends with Tenon's capsule, which attaches firmly to the limbus. The conjunctiva is a highly vascular, delicate tissue containing many mucous-secreting goblet cells. The vascularity and mobility of the conjunctiva can be used to the surgeon's advantage to act as a graft for corneal defects. The conjunctiva is also a site of localization of lymphocytes and provides a reservoir of immunocompetent cells for the globe, in particular the avascular cornea.

The *third eyelid* is a mobile, semirigid structure located inferionasal to the globe (Figure 1-1). It is covered on both palpe-

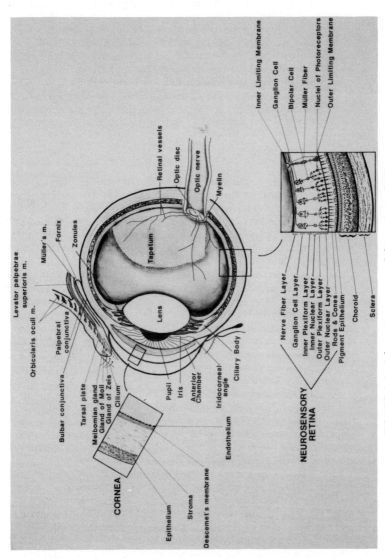

FIGURE 1-2. Schematic anatomy of the canine and feline eye.

5

bral and bulbar surfaces by conjunctiva. The third eyelid owes its rigidity to a T-shaped piece of hyaline cartilage located within its substantia propria. At the base of the cartilage is a seromucoid lacrimal gland that produces approximately one third of the precorneal tear film. Poorly defined connective tissue attaches the gland and base of the cartilage to the sclera and periorbita inferiorly. Spontaneous breakdown of these attachments with prolapse of the gland occurs not uncommonly, particularly in the American Cocker Spaniel and English Bulldog breeds. Removal of the gland in such cases is contraindicated as it may predispose to future development of keratoconjunctivitis sicca; the gland should be repositioned and sutured in place as described in Chapter 5.

Cornea

The *cornea* is the transparent, avascular anterior portion of the outer fibrous coat of the eye (Figure 1-2). The cornea consists of surface epithelium, collagenous stroma, and Descemet's membrane, which is the basement membrane produced by the inner endothelial monolayer. As the cornea is avascular, its oxygen and nutritional needs are met by diffusion externally from the precorneal tear film and internally from the aqueous humor; the peripheral cornea is also oxygenated by the limbal capillary plexus. Corneal transparency is a product of several factors unique to corneal physiology. Relative dehydration of the cornea is maintained by an active Na^+-K^+ ATPase-associated pump mechanism within the endothelial monolayer. The regular arrangement of the collagen fibrils in the corneal stroma minimizes scattered light and thus enhances transparency. The normal absence of pigment and blood vessels in the stroma is also a requirement for optical transparency.

The cornea has remarkable healing capabilities. Simple epithelial defects are covered by a combination of sliding of adjacent cells and mitosis to restore normal cell number. Wounds that extend into the stroma heal first by re-epithelialization, with a longer period of time required to fill the stromal defect. Corneal scarring is a result of the irregular pattern created by replacement collagen fibrils. Vascularization is expected to accompany any corneal injury or inflammatory condition that persists longer than seven to ten days and contributes to the opaque granulation tissue that initially fills a deep corneal wound. Descemet's membrane is elastic and tends to resist tearing during an injury. Wounds extending to Descemet's membrane (descemetocele) and full-thickness lacerations are indications for immediate surgical management. Some reparative properties are attributed to the canine endothelium, little to the feline.

Iris and Ciliary Body

The iris and ciliary body comprise the anterior portion of the middle, vascular coat of the eye, called the *uvea* (Figure 1-2). The iris creates a pupillary opening of variable diameter to adjust the quantity of light that is able to pass through the lens to reach the photosensitive retina. This variable aperture is maintained by the sympathetically supplied radial dilator muscle and the parasympathetically supplied circumferential sphincter muscle. Both muscles are located on the posterior side of the iris, deep to the pigmented epithelial layer. The iris anterior to these muscles consists of a loose, vascular connective tissue that is variably pigmented. Full-thickness corneal wounds often seal with iris tissue, which must be replaced into the anterior chamber (if viable) or excised. Surgical manipulations of the iris are frequently accompanied by hemorrhage that may complicate postoperative healing. Electrocautery may be used to control hemorrhage.

The *ciliary body* is the posterior continuation of the iris and consists of an anterior portion called the *pars plicata* (with the ciliary processes) and a posterior portion called the *pars plana*. The ciliary body is covered throughout by a bilayered epithelium of which only the deeper layer is pigmented. Aqueous humor is produced by the ciliary epithelium through a combination of passive ultrafiltration and active secretion involving carbonic anhydrase. The passive production of aqueous humor is influenced by mean arterial blood pressure. Inflammation of the anterior uvea will result in reduced active aqueous secretion and thus lowered intraocular pressure. The stroma of the ciliary body contains the smooth fibers of the parasympathetically innervated ciliary muscle, which is important in accommodation of the lens for near vision.

Aqueous humor circulates from the ciliary processes in the posterior chamber of the eye, through the pupil, to exit via the trabecular meshwork of the iridocorneal angle. During this process, metabolites are exchanged with the avascular lens and cornea. Morphologic or physiologic barriers to aqueous circulation and outflow are responsible for elevations in intraocular pressure (glaucoma).

Lens

The *lens* is a transparent, biconvex structure anchored equatorially to the ciliary body by collagenous zonule fibers (Figure 1-2). Contraction of the ciliary muscle alters the degree of curvature of the lens, thereby changing its optical power. The lens is surrounded by an outer capsule; deep to the anterior portion of the capsule is a monolayer of cuboidal epithelium. These epithelial cells are metabolically very active and undergo mitosis throughout life. As the cells multiply they move to the equator of the lens, where they elongate and gradually lose their nucleus and other organelles to form the spindle-shaped lens fibers. These fibers are added in a circumferential arrangement so that older fibers are within the deeper portion of the lens. The fiber ends meet anteriorly at the upright Y suture and posteriorly at the inverted Y suture.

The anterior epithelial cells utilize glucose, which diffuses into the lens from the circulating aqueous humor and is broken down anaerobically to lactic acid. Saturation of the normal pathways for glucose metabolism occurs in diabetes mellitus and results in accumulation of sorbitol within the lens. Sorbitol attracts water, which results in a clinically observable cataract that usually progresses rapidly.

Retina

The *retina* is a complex photosensory structure consisting of ten layers: (1) pigment epithelium, (2) photoreceptors (rod and cone outer segments), (3) external limiting membrane (Müller cell processes), (4) outer nuclear layer (photoreceptor nuclei), (5) outer plexiform layer, (6) inner nuclear layer (nuclei of Müller, amacrine, horizontal, and bipolar cells), (7) inner plexiform layer, (8) ganglion cell layer, (9) nerve fiber layer (axons of ganglion cells), and (10) inner limiting membrane (Müller cell processes) (Figure 1–2). The principal neuronal connections of the retina involve the photoreceptors, which synapse with the ganglion cells in the inner plexiform layer. The axons of the ganglion cells form the nerve fiber layer and join to make up the optic nerve at the posterior pole. The amacrine and horizontal cells form internal connections between bipolar cells and may thus exert a regulatory influence. Müller cells are a nonneuronal constituent that forms a supporting matrix and the barriers of the inner and outer limiting membranes.

Inherited retinal degenerative processes initially involve the photoreceptors, either rods, cones, or both. With time the condition usually progresses to involve the other retinal layers, and diffuse thinning and blindness results.

Tapetum

The *tapetum* is a modification of the choroid located deep to the neural retina. It is composed of a highly organized arrangement of crystals containing zinc and riboflavin, which results in a reflective appearance. The color of the tapetum ranges from green to blue to yellow and varies with the species, breed, and age. Thinning of the overlying retina (as occurs in retinal degeneration) results in a hyperreflective appearance of the tapetum.

Optic Nerve and Central Visual Pathways

The optic nerve consists of combined axons of the ganglion cells and is surrounded by all three meningeal layers of the central nervous system. The optic disk is the origin of the optic nerve within the globe; its irregular triangular appearance is a result of the variable quantity of myelin surrounding the optic nerve (Figure 1–2). The optic nerve exits the orbit at the optic foramen. The right and left optic nerves meet at the optic chiasm, located rostral to the pituitary gland. In domestic animals, the majority (sixty-five to seventy-five percent) of nerve fibers cross in the chiasm to travel as the optic tracts to the contralateral geniculate nucleus. This decussation is responsible for coordinated bilateral vision as well as the occurrence of a consensual pupillary light response (Figure 1–3).

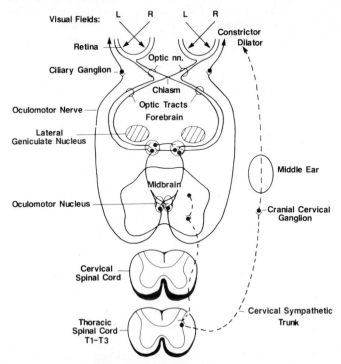

FIGURE 1–3. Pupillary pathways.

The majority of axons in the optic tracts terminate in the lateral geniculate nucleus, synapsing on neurons whose axons form the optic radiations and terminate in the occipital cortex. This pathway is responsible for conscious visual perception.

The remaining optic tract axons bypass the lateral geniculate nucleus and terminate in the rostral colliculus of the pretectal area. Parasympathetic axons originating here synapse in the oculomotor nucleus of the midbrain, origin of the oculomotor nerves, whose axons synapse in the ciliary ganglion prior to entering the globe as the short ciliary nerves to the pupillary sphincter muscles. This pathway is responsible for the direct and consensual pupillary light responses.

Sympathetic control of the pupillary dilator muscle originates in the hypothalamus with preganglionic neurons in the first four segments of the thoracic spinal cord. These axons join the sympathetic trunk terminating in the cranial cervical ganglion. Postganglionic fibers travel to the eye with the internal carotid artery to join the ophthalmic nerve and are distributed to the ciliary muscle, pupillary dilator, third eyelid, and the Müller's muscle of the upper lid. Compromise of sympathetic innervation to the globe results in the classic signs of Horner's syndrome: ptosis (drooping of the upper lid), miosis (pupillary constriction), and protrusion of the third eyelid.

2 | *Diagnostics*

Dennis Hacker

INSTRUMENTATION

Although some veterinary clinicians feel competent in the field of ophthalmology, others admit to having a paucity of basic understanding in the area, so before discussing specific techniques of ocular examination, a brief description of instrumentation is appropriate. Part of the mystique that surrounds clinical ophthalmology is the misassumption that accurate diagnostics require an examination room full of expensive equipment that can be mastered only with specialized training. Quite to the contrary, the vast majority of ophthalmic conditions can be diagnosed with a few relatively inexpensive tools and techniques that almost every practitioner can learn with a bit of practice.

Direct Ophthalmoscope

The ophthalmoscope is used for high-magnification examination of specific lesions, primarily of the ocular fundus. The direct ophthalmoscope has a focus wheel with lenses which vary in diopter power from +40 D (black) to −25 D (red). The choice of Welch Allyn,[a] Propper,[b] or other scope is determined by personal preference and/or cost. This equipment may be wall-mounted or portable. The basic set should also include a veterinary otoscope. Useful attachments for an ophthalmoscope are a Finhoff transilluminator and a cobalt blue filter.

Maximal pupillary dilation with topical 1.0% tropicamide is essential for thorough ophthalmoscopy in the dog and cat. The most expeditious way to use the ophthalmoscope is to set the focus wheel to +15, using the large spot aperture; working at arm's length from the patient, visualize the patient's fundic reflex while both of the examiner's eyes are open. This is an excellent method

---

a. Welch Allyn, Skaneateles Falls, NY.
b. Propper Manufacturing Co., Inc., Long Island City, NY.

to compare pupil size from one eye to the other. Lesions anywhere in the cornea, anterior or posterior chamber, lens, or vitreous manifest as defects in the fundic reflex. Next, set the focus wheel to 0 and move toward the patient until the fundus is clearly seen. Use your right eye to examine the patient's right eye and your left eye to examine the patient's left eye. In this manner, the ophthalmoscope is between the patient (teeth!) and the examiner (nose and ears!). Once you are within one to two inches of the patient, with both of your eyes open, turn the focus wheel to obtain the best focus of the fundus. If a lesion in question is elevated from the fundus into the vitreous space, more positive (black) diopters will be needed to bring the lesion into focus. If a lesion is, for example, a pit in the optic nerve or choroid, more negative (red) diopters will be needed to focus on the lesion.

The transilluminator provides a light source for external eye and pupillary light examinations. With the cobalt blue filter, fluorescence of fluorescein-stained ulcers can easily be seen. The diagnostic otoscopic head may be used if the practitioner desires magnification of lesions seen on the external examination.

Hand Lens

Due to the narrow field of view and great magnification (14x–16x) afforded by direct ophthalmoscopy, doing a thorough examination of a patient's fundus is very difficult. The most expeditious screening examination of the fundus is accomplished by using an inexpensive hand lens. Nikon and Volk lenses are excellent, but their prices may make them impractical for the clinical practitioner. A reasonable compromise is a Macro +10 to +20 camera filter manufactured by various companies. Many camera stores can order these lenses, which come in various sizes; I would suggest getting a filter approximately 30 to 55 mm in diameter.

To use the hand lens, start at arm's length from the patient holding your transilluminator in front of your nose and aimed at the patient's cornea; you should get a good tapetal or fundic reflection. Then position the lens in front of the patient's eye, parallel to your own eye. The best view usually occurs with the lens between two and four inches in front of the patient's cornea, depending on the lens focal length. Move the lens toward or away from the cornea until the entire lens is filled with the fundus image. To steady the lens, rest your fingers on the patient's frontal or nasal area. Hold the lens with the left hand to examine the patient's right eye and with the right hand to view the patient's left eye. Keep both eyes open and use the light directly in front of the examiner's nose to produce a binocular image. Practice is essential to gain expertise.

Schiötz Tonometer

Accurate estimation of intraocular pressure (IOP) is impossible by using one's fingers because subtle changes in IOP are imperceptible with this crude technique. Although applanation tonometry is quite accurate, the equipment is very expensive. An indentation (Schiötz) tonometer is an acceptable and economical alternative in a small animal practice. To ensure accuracy, the instrument should be standardized or calibrated, and a certificate indicating accuracy should accompany the instrument.

Topical anesthesia is needed before tonometry is performed; either proparacaine[c] or tetracaine[d] is acceptable. One drop of anesthetic in each eye approximately twenty seconds prior to tonometry provides adequate corneal anesthesia.

Prior to each use, the tonometer should be checked for accuracy and to assure ease of operation. Hold the tonometer by the finger-holding bracket and place the corneal footplate on the steel footpad provided in the case. After you obtain a tonometer reading of zero, the patient should be seated with its nose elevated toward the ceiling so that the cornea is parallel with the examination table. No pressure should be applied to the neck because jugular vein occlusion may result in erroneously elevated IOP. If the patient cannot be held in this manner, or if the patient is obese and jugular collapse occurs upon head elevation, the patient can be rolled onto its back and the nose held perpendicular to and the cornea parallel to the examination table surface. Once the patient is restrained, retract the eyelids in such a manner that no pressure is applied to the globe. Apply the corneal footplate to the cornea and lower the finger-holding bracket so that the tonometer is free-floating, that is, between the top and bottom stops. If the third eyelid covers part of the cornea, the footplate should be gently directed under the third eyelid. Allow the tonometer to rest only long enough to get a stable reading. Then raise it slightly off the corneal surface and repeat the process to obtain two more readings. The human conversion tables that come with the instrument underestimate IOP in the dog and cat due to species differences in anatomy. A table for conversion of scale readings to estimated IOP is available for the canine eye; "normal" values for the dog and cat are in the range of 20 to 30 mm Hg (Table 2-1). The 7.5 gm weight is the weight I routinely use. For a practical assessment, I take the value of the weight used ± 2.5 scale

c. Ophthetic, Allergan Pharmaceuticals, Inc., Irvine, CA; Alcaine, Alcon Laboratories, Inc., Fort Worth, TX.

d. Tetracaine HCl, Pharmafair, Inc., Hauppauge, NY.

TABLE 2–1. Schiötz Conversion Table for the Canine Eye.

SCHIÖTZ SCALE READING	IOP (MM HG) 5.5 G WT	IOP (MM HG) 7.5 G WT	IOP (MM HG) 10.0 G WT
0	56	76	99
1	49	67	88
2	43	59	79
3	38	53	70
4	34	47	62
5	30	42	55
6	27	37	49
7	24	33	44
8	22	30	40
9	20	27	36
10	19	25	32
11	17	23	29
12	17	21	27
13	16	20	24
14	<16	19	23
15		18	21
16		<18	20
17			19
18			<19

From Peiffer, R.L., Calibration of the Schiötz Tonometer for the Normal Canine Eye. *Amer. J. Vet. Res.* 38:1881–1889, 1977.

units to be the normal IOP range. Therefore, for the 5.0 gm weight, a scale reading of 2.5 to 7.5 is within normal IOP range. If the scale reading is lower than 2.5, the IOP is elevated (remember that steel = 0). Readings higher than 7.5 indicate lower than usual IOP and are suggestive of uveitis. With the 7.5 gm weight, normal readings are from 5.0 to 10.0. The tonometer footplate and indentation rod should be cleaned with alcohol between patients to minimize the chances of spreading ocular pathogens. When necessary, disassemble the instrument and use a pipe cleaner to clean the center bore of the tonometer to allow smooth and reliable operation.

Schirmer Tear Test Strips

Although #41 Whatman filter paper can be cut and used to assess tear function, both for convenience and for sterility, Schirmer tear test (STT) strips[e] are superior. They come in a box of twenty-five large envelopes with ten strips per envelope, sealed two per individual pouch. The test measures the production of

e. Alcon Laboratories, Inc., Fort Worth, TX.

the aqueous portion of the tear film and is extremely helpful in diagnosing keratoconjunctivitis sicca (KCS). These strips absorb any aqueous fluid in the conjunctival cul-de-sac.

The strips should be folded at the notch while in the pouch to prevent any oils that may be on the fingers from contaminating the tip. Remove excess mucus from the eye and adnexa using dry, cotton-tipped applicators or cotton balls. No fluids should be placed on the eye immediately prior to testing, as erroneously elevated STT values will result. If any fluid has been inadvertently introduced onto the eye, the adnexa should be dried with cotton gauze or cotton balls and ten to fifteen minutes allowed to pass prior to starting the STT; this precaution allows excess fluid to exit the conjunctival cul-de-sac via the nasolacrimal system and by evaporation. If you have any doubt concerning the validity of the test, repeat it after a few minutes delay. A topical anesthetic placed on the eye results in a lowered STT value due to inhibition of reflex lacrimation. Evert the lower eyelid of the patient with your thumb, and place the notched end of the test strip behind the nasal one-third of the lid. Return the eyelid to the normal position, and hold the eyelids closed, if necessary, to retain the strip. After one minute, place the strip directly on the scale of the package and obtain the STT value. By placing the strip on the scale rather than adjacent to it, a more precise STT value is obtained.

In the dog with clinical signs, STT values of 5 mm or less within one minute are diagnostic for dry eye. Values of 5 to 10 mm are suspicious, and values greater than 10 mm are considered normal. Although cats may have "normal" values as low as 3 to 6 mm/min, their mean values are considered similar to the dog. Always interpret these values in conjunction with the clinical signs; we diagnose and treat disease, not numbers. In any patient with clinical signs, STT values less than 5 mm/min are diagnostic for KCS.

Ophthalmic Stains

Fluorescein stain is indispensable in a clinical practice. As it is lipophobic and hydrophilic, this agent will not stain the corneal epithelium, which is lipid in composition. If the epithelium is absent, as in an ulcer, the stroma, which is freely permeable to aqueous solutions, will retain fluorescein. Fluorescein may be purchased in the form of ophthalmic drops, but because bacterial growth may occur in the fluid if it is used inappropriately, the stain used in clinical practices should be in the form of sterile strips.[f] When using the strips, no fluid need be added to the strip

---

f. Fluor-I-Strip[R], Ayerst Laboratories, New York, NY.

unless the patient has low tear production; adding fluid to the strip will overstain the eye and may cause confusion as to the true lesion. Simply elevate the upper eyelid and gently touch the strip to the bulbar conjunctiva. If you are able to see *any* moisture on the strip after you lift it off the conjunctiva, more than enough stain should be on the eye. To be sure, use your transilluminator with the cobalt blue filter to see if the tear film at the margin of the lower eyelid is stained. Tear or snip off the used end of the strip and stain the second eye as with the first.

Rose bengal stain is optional in a clinical practice, but it is useful to stain mucus and devitalized epithelium. Typically, it comes as a 1.0% solution[g] or impregnated on sterile strips.[h] If the solution is used, it may be diluted 1:1 with an equal amount of sterile saline to minimize the irritation caused by the 1.0% concentration. If the strips are used, wet the ends of these strips with collyrium to ensure that an adequate amount of stain is available. In either case, place one drop of stain on the cornea of each eye, wait one minute, and rinse liberally with collyrium. Topical anesthetics, if applied to the eye prior to use of rose bengal stain, will cause the surface to become irregular; the stain will be retained by the epithelium and may be interpreted erroneously as a corneal abnormality.

Magnification and Illumination

Magnification, essential when examining or performing surgery on the eye, can be obtained with an Optivisor[i] or with ophthalmic loupes. The low cost, comfort, and ease of use of the Optivisor make it versatile in practice.

While you are using magnification, a hands-free light source is helpful. A technician can provide this using a transilluminator, but this approach is somewhat labor-intensive. A more efficacious method is to purchase a headlight,[j] which can be focused right where you are looking. A headlight is also helpful in ophthalmic surgery when you are working very close to the surgical site.

The biomicroscope is the ultimate instrument of controlled magnification and illumination. Expense limits their availability in a general practice but a slitlamp is an invaluable and essential tool for someone with a serious interest in ophthalmology.

---

g. Rose bengal 1%, Akorn, Inc., Abita Springs, LA.
h. Barnes-Hind, Inc., Sunnyvale, CA.
i. Donegan Optical Co., Lenexa, KS.
j. Welch Allyn, Skaneateles Falls, NY.

Lacrimal Cannula

A 23-gauge, curved lacrimal cannula[k] is useful for flushing the dog's nasolacrimal system. A homemade cannula for cats can be made by filing the point of a 25-gauge hypodermic needle flat, reaming out the new tip using the point of a #11 scalpel blade, and finally using emory paper or steel wool to smooth the tip. Prior to use, the cannula should be flushed with fluid to assess patency and clean the bore.

Flushing the nasolacrimal system is done after topically anesthetizing the eye and restraining the patient; sedation or anesthesia may be occasionally required, especially in cats. Place the cannula on a 3-ml syringe containing 1 to 2 ml of an appropriate fluid (I use tap water). Place the index finger or thumb on the plunger of the syringe and gently insert the cannula into the upper lacrimal punctum. By gently directing the cannula tip medially and simultaneously moving the syringe toward the dorsal midline of the patient's head, the cannula should drop into the lacrimal sac. In the normal dog or cat, flushing with the cannula in the lacrimal sac should cause little or no resistance. As fluid comes from the lower punctum, digital occlusion of the lower punctum will then force fluid through the nasolacrimal duct. Fluid or bubbles may then come from the nares, or the patient may cough or swallow. If resistance is encountered, either the cannula is not in the lacrimal sac or an obstruction may be present. In this case, referral to an ophthalmologist is recommended for diagnostic radiography and/or cannulation of the nasolacrimal system.

Sterile Swabs and Spatula

To obtain material for a culture from any ocular surface, a dry, sterile swab should be wetted with sterile saline *prior* to culturing; many more isolates are obtained with a wet swab than a dry swab. Swabs can also be used mechanically to debride ulcers around which loose epithelium is revealed by fluorescein staining. A metal spatula, sterilizable by flame, will provide equal or superior samples for microbiology and/or cytology.

Mydriatic

To facilitate a thorough examination of the lens and posterior segment, the pupil should be adequately dilated. A mydriatic

---

k. Becton, Dickinson and Co., Rutherford, NJ.

and/or cycloplegic can be used. Tropicamide,[1] due to its speed of onset, relative freedom of side effects, and short duration of action, is superior for diagnostic work. Maximum mydriasis with this parasympatholytic occurs within fifteen to twenty minutes after one drop is applied to the eye and lasts for several hours.

Forceps

Good quality Bishop-Harmon forceps are excellent for general ophthalmic use. Forceps without teeth (for grasping corneal/conjunctival foreign bodies) and with 0.3-mm teeth (for examining the conjunctiva and third eyelid) are recommended. Prior to the use of forceps, several drops of topical anesthetic should be applied to the eye. When grasping the third eyelid, care should be exercised *not* to grasp the nictitans structure by its full thickness. Topical anesthesia will not fully anesthetize deeper structures and pain will be evoked in grasping the third eyelid in this manner. Grasp only the palpebral (anterior) surface and lift the third eyelid to examine both sides.

EXAMINATION TECHNIQUE

Ocular examinations often are not conducted routinely in a busy veterinary practice. One reason often given is that a physical and complete ophthalmic exam prolong an office visit. Not so! By using a modification of the traditional protocol, a thorough ophthalmic and physical examination may be conducted effectively and efficiently. Figure 2–1 is a flowchart that may be useful as a guide for performing such a physical and ophthalmic exam. Portions of this exam may be deleted as desired or as practical, considering the situation. The elements of a general ophthalmic examination are described below.

Prior to beginning the examination, the clinician must ascertain the chief ocular complaint for which the patient has been presented for evaluation. A prolonged history is postponed until after pupillary responses are checked and the mydriatic is instilled. During the fifteen to twenty minutes required for the mydriatic to take effect, the history and a physical examination are conducted.

The examination should commence in a dimly lit room. First, the patient should be viewed sagitally at about arm's length. Using a penlight, a transilluminator, or a direct ophthalmoscope (as to visualize a bilateral fundic or tapetal reflex), obtain information about pupil size of each eye and the transparency of ocular media.

---

1. Mydriacyl, Alcon Laboratories, Inc., Fort Worth, TX.

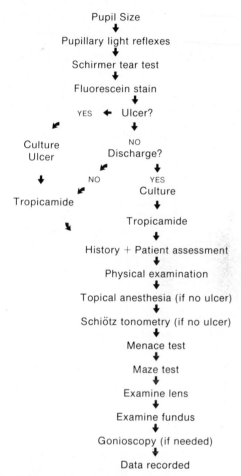

FIGURE 2-1. Flowchart for ophthalmic examination.

The pupillary light reflex (PLR) is next assessed. First, each eye is directly stimulated, with the light source held 2 to 5 cm from the patient's eye. The light beam is directed down the optic axis of each globe, and the completeness and briskness of the PLR is noted, in turn, for each eye. The response of the unstimulated eye is noted as the consensual reflex of the stimulated eye. In the normal patient, both pupils respond when either eye is stimulated, although the pupil of the consensual eye may not constrict to exactly the same size as the pupil of the stimulated eye. When the light source is rapidly moved to the previously unstimulated eye, further slight pupillary constriction may be observed.

The ocular adnexa, cornea, and conjunctiva should be examined with direct and oblique illumination. Symmetry and normalcy of adnexa should be assessed. Palpate the eyelids and orbital margin, gently retropulsing the globes into the orbit. Color of the conjunctiva, prominence of conjunctival and scleral blood vessels, and character of the conjunctiva should be noted. The corneal transparency, surface smoothness, continuity, and luster should be evaluated. The character and quantity of any ocular discharge should be noted.

The Schirmer tear test should be performed prior to the institution of any medication or fluid. As the strips are sterile, they will not alter any subsequent bacterial or fungal culture result. This test is indicated on any patient with a mucoid or purulent ocular discharge and/or chronic external ocular disease.

Fluorescein staining is warranted when there is evidence of corneal discontinuity (ulcer) or haziness, or in any painful eye for which a cause for the pain is not evident. Fluorescein strips are sterile and will not alter forthcoming culture results.

Severe corneal ulcers, conjunctivitis unresponsive to treatment, or eyes with purulent ocular discharge should be cultured for both bacteria and fungi. A sterile swab, wetted with sterile saline or collyrium, a prepackaged culture swab,[m] or a heat-sterilized spatula may be used. Swabs should be discarded if they touch facial or eyelid hairs. Culture results tend to be more accurate when immediate inoculation is performed, but in a clinical practice this may not be possible. If immediate inoculation of culture media is not possible, then a stat pickup from a laboratory should be requested, and the sample should be refrigerated or kept cool until picked up.

Because pupillary dilation is necessary for the remainder of the ophthalmic exam, one drop of tropicamide should be applied to each eye. If more than one drop is used, both eyes should receive the same amount; equal dilation will then become a diagnostic parameter.

The patient's history should now be taken while the pupils are dilating. Often, clients will attempt to assist you by trying to give the patient's entire life story. Alternatively, they may not present events in a chronological order, causing great confusion in their minds as well as yours. I have found it helpful to ask specific questions to elicit a concise history. A written autohistory may be used; however, I feel these should be followed with verbal confirmation of information given. Questions should elicit the

---

m. Culturette, Marion Laboratories, Inc., Kansas City, MO.

client's opinion of the quality of the patient's vision. The nature of the ocular problem, its duration, the initiating complaint, any systemic or topical medications used, the patient's general health, and the ocular and general health status of other household pets should be elucidated. Vaccination status and diet history also are helpful. Finally, ask the client if he or she wants to tell you anything else about this condition. Quite often, the client has a significant insight into the problem, but is intimidated into silence without this question.

As the history is taken or confirmed, another important portion of the exam may be conducted by observing the patient for willingness to move about, a tendency to bump into objects, or attempts to rub or paw at the eye(s) or hold the eye(s) closed.

A general physical examination is an important aspect of the ophthalmic evaluation. Temperature, pulse, respiration, and information gathered from an oral examination and lymph node and abdominal palpation may assist your diagnosis. Tractability and mentation of the patient may be evaluated.

Intraocular tension readings of domestic small animals are now obtained with the Schiötz tonometer as previously described. Schiötz tonometry should not be performed on an eye with a deep corneal ulcer, as corneal perforation could result! When a corneal ulcer exists and elevated IOP is suspected, referral to a veterinary ophthalmologist is suggested.

The anterior chamber should be evaluated for depth and clarity. The contents of the normal anterior chamber do not disperse light. Intraocular inflammation disrupts the blood-aqueous barrier and allows protein access to the aqueous humor. This higher than normal concentration of protein causes scattering of light (flare), making a light beam visible as it passes through the anterior chamber. Aqueous flare may be evaluated by using the slit or small spot aperture light beam of the direct ophthalmoscope to direct the light beam through the anterior chamber at an oblique angle. The clinician should be aware, however, that a slit lamp is necessary to detect subtle aqueous flare, and referral to a veterinary ophthalmologist may be warranted. Material such as blood (hyphema) or purulent exudate (hypopyon) indicate significant intraocular abnormalities.

The iris should be examined with both direct and retroillumination. This need not await pupillary dilation. An iris surface that is redder than normal may be caused by neovascularization (rubeosis iridis), hemorrhage, or venous congestion. A darker iris than usual may indicate increased natural pigment (melanin) or ocular disease. Retroillumination is obtained by aiming the light source through the pupil to get a fundic or tapetal reflex. Iris atrophy can be recognized as thin spots, often at the pupillary margin, that appear brighter than adjacent normal iris.

While awaiting the pupillary dilation, the menace reflex, which can give some indication as to the vision of the patient, can be evaluated. A direct poking motion at the patient, while using a plastic shield to prevent response to air movement, may be used. Alternatively, a rapid vertical movement of the clinician's hand through the patient's visual axis (without causing air movement toward the patient's eye) may be used. Occasionally normal cats or dogs do not menace with these techniques.

By the time all of the steps described above are taken, the pupil should be dilated. If dilation has not occurred and the IOP is low, uveitis should be suspected. A maze test should be conducted in a brightly lit room with white light (photopic conditions) and in dim red-filtered or very dim white light (scotopic conditions). A simple maze can be constructed with a trash can and a stool as obstacles. The client should stand to one side of these obstructions and call the patient only once. The patient should be observed for ability to traverse the maze without bumping into objects. Successful navigation, bumped objects, or reluctance to move should be noted. If a monocular visual deficit is suspected, each eye may be alternately occluded, using gauze squares and tape, and the maze run several times.

When the previously instilled mydriatic has caused complete pupillary dilation, the lens and ocular fundus may be critically evaluated. The lens may be examined initially with a penlight or transilluminator. Alternatively, the slit beam aperture of the direct ophthalmoscope may be used. In either event, external magnification will aid critical examination. The slit beam allows localization of any lesions within the light beam. An alternative method of lesion localization is achieved by observing the apparent motion of a lesion with movement of either the patient's eye or movement of the observer. If, for example, the clinician moves nasally, as the patient's eye remains stationary, lesions in the anterior lens will appear to move laterally. A lesion in the posterior portion of the lens will appear to move nasally. Alternatively, if the clinician remains stationary and the patient moves its eye in either direction, anterior lens lesions will appear to move with the eye movement and posterior lesions will appear to move opposite the direction of ocular movement. Appearance and location of any lesions seen should be noted.

The fundus should now be evaluated using the hand-held lens as previously described. A transilluminator or a penlight may be used as a light source. Any lesion seen using the hand-lens may be critically evaluated using the direct ophthalmoscope.

Gonioscopy is not often done by the clinical veterinarian. This is a fairly difficult procedure, requiring expensive lenses, and the procedure may not be performed frequently enough to maintain proficiency. If gonioscopy is to be done, it should be done last in the examination because gonioscopic-prism solutions alter the corneal surface and the tear film and make examining the ocular fundus difficult.

Information obtained during all portions of the examination should be recorded in the patient's permanent record to give the basis for diagnosis or consultation with a veterinary ophthalmologist. The information also makes referral to this or other ophthalmologic texts easier.

3 | *Therapeutics*

Dennis Hacker

INTRODUCTION

The great majority of ophthalmic conditions can be adequately managed with a small selection of pharmaceuticals. For common conditions such as bacterial or allergic conjunctivitis, anterior uveitis, keratoconjunctivitis sicca, or corneal ulcers, or for emergencies such as acute glaucoma, the practitioner should have an appropriate armamentarium of medications available. More expensive and/or less commonly utilized agents are more efficiently dispensed by prescription through a pharmacy.

Successful management of ophthalmic cases depends on: an accurate diagnosis; selection of medication(s) that is efficacious for the diagnosed condition; and getting the medication to the desired tissues in therapeutic levels adequate to resolve the diagnosed condition. Failure of a case to respond may be related to inadequacies of any of the above principles or to the severity or refractory nature of the disease process, for example, a fulminating endophthalmitis or glaucoma. Because in ophthalmic cases rapidity of disease control is frequently related to the ultimate visual outcome, patients require regular follow-up examinations as dictated by the severity of the condition. Nonresponsive cases require reconfirmation of the diagnosis and/or thoughtful alteration of the selected therapeutic regimen.

Ophthalmic drugs may be divided into a few groups based upon desired therapeutic effects: antimicrobials; anti-inflammatory agents; autonomic agents; and ocular hypotensive agents. The latter two categories overlap, as some autonomic agents not only control pupillary size but affect intraocular pressure as well.

Ophthalmic drugs may be given by systemic means, either orally or parenterally; by local injection (subconjunctival injection); or by topical administration. In general, the route of administration will depend upon the location and severity of the disease process. The majority of adnexal and corneal diseases are adequately treated with local and/or topically applied medication to achieve an adequate therapeutic level of medication in tissues. Posterior segment, optic nerve, and orbital disease are best managed with systemic medication, as topically or locally applied medication will in general not achieve therapeutic levels in these structures.

ORAL DRUGS

Oral medications to be used for ophthalmic cases include antibiotics, anti-inflammatory agents, and antiglaucoma medications, consisting of carbonic anhydrase inhibitors and glycerin.

Antimicrobials

Most practices have a supply of trimethoprim-sulfa drugs[a] and chloramphenicol.[b] These drugs are excellent if required for postoperative and postinjury prophylaxis and for treating ocular and periocular bacterial infections resulting from injury. In my experience, the most common infectious bacterial agents are *Staphylococcus* and *Streptococcus* spp., which are commonly sensitive to these drugs. The sensitivity of these bacteria is not always the same in a referral practice in which most cases have been treated previously with other drugs; in this situation, culture and sensitivity tests are frequently performed during the initial examination. Amoxicillin drops,[c] a penicillin analog, are very convenient and in my experience have been effective for treating cats and kittens. When resistant organisms are isolated via bacterial culture, other antibiotics may be prescribed through a pharmacy as indicated by the individual sensitivity.

Anti-Inflammatory Agents

The oral anti-inflammatory drugs of choice, used for control of intraocular and extraocular inflammation, are the corticosteroids prednisolone and prednisone and the nonsteroidal anti-inflammatory drugs (NSAIDS) aspirin and flunixin meglumine.[d] The most commonly used corticosteroid in human medicine ophthalmology is prednisone, which is available in tablets in strengths ranging from 5 to 50 mg. The most common form used in veterinary medicine is prednisolone (5 mg only). The difference

---

a. Ditrim tablets and injectable, Syntex Animal Health, Inc., West Des Moines, IA; Tribrissen, Burroughs Wellcome Co., Research Triangle Park, NC.

b. Chloromycetin, Kapseals and Palmitate, Parke-Davis, Morris Plains, NJ.

c. Amoxidrops, Beecham Laboratories, Bristol, TN.

d. Banamine, Schering Corporation, Kenilworth, NJ.

in these medications is that prednisone must be activated by the liver to form prednisolone, the biologically active form. For mild intraocular or extraocular inflammation, 0.1 to 0.25 mg/kg of either may be all that is needed. For severe intraocular or retrobulbar inflammation, 0.5 to 1.0 mg/kg or more may be required. Although dexamethasone is frequently prescribed in clinical practices, I feel that the short-acting prednisone-type drugs give excellent anti-inflammatory effects and have a shorter half-life, which is of value if an error in judgment is made concerning when to use steroids. Prednisone-type drugs are virtually eliminated from the body within 24 hours, whereas dexamethasone and other halogen-substituted corticosteroids have a 48-hour or longer elimination time span. The NSAIDs inhibit the cyclo-oxygenase enzyme and therefore block the production of inflammation-causing prostaglandins. Flunixin meglumine, a potent anti-inflammatory agent, is occasionally used in dogs. Dogs occasionally develop gastrointestinal bleeding or kidney problems from prolonged or high-dosage treatment. I have used flunixin at a rate of 0.5 mg/kg once daily (QD) for three days only in the dog. In the dog, aspirin dosage rates vary but a dosage of 15 to 25 mg/kg of buffered aspirin BID to TID seems to be well tolerated. Fecal occult blood examinations should occasionally be performed on all patients when these agents are given for a prolonged period of time.

Ocular Hypotensive Agents

Carbonic anhydrase inhibitors (CAI) are used in the treatment of acute glaucoma to reduce the quantity of aqueous humor that is produced. The CAI of choice in small animal practice is dichlorphenamide.[e] It appears to be reasonably well tolerated by most patients and causes little gastric or metabolic upset if dosed at the rate of 2 to 5 mg/kg BID to TID. This medication is not routinely stocked in all human pharmacies, and the client may have to wait for the medication to be ordered or may have to check at several pharmacies. An alternative is methazolamide,[f] which will be found in virtually all pharmacies and is dosed at the rate of 5 to 10 mg/kg BID to TID. These medications are expensive and associated with the side effects of metabolic acidosis and hypokalemia; common symptoms of toxicity are restlessness, hyperventilation, and vomiting. Because of these side effects, the expense of the medication, and the poor long-term

e. Daranide, Merck Sharp & Dohme, West Point, PA.
f. Neptazane, Lederle Laboratories, Wayne, NJ.

control of intraocular pressure in our patients, we recommend surgical alternatives in the long-term control of glaucoma.

Glycerin is an oral hyperosmotic agent used in treating glaucoma. It may, through dehydration, reduce the amount of aqueous humor produced. Glycerin draws fluid from the extracellular space and thus reduces the vitreous humor volume. It is readily available and can be acquired in strengths of 50 to 90%. The dosage rate is variable and is usually given at 1.0 to 2.0 g/kg. Glycerine may be mixed with chocolate milk and will be consumed readily by small animal patients. When giving hyperosmotic agents, water should be withheld for several hours after dosing to allow fluid to be removed from the extracellular space.

Giving oral medications is usually inadvisable if surgery is anticipated; if surgery is anticipated in a patient with acute glaucoma, glycerin would be contraindicated.

INJECTABLE DRUGS

Antimicrobials

The routine injectable antibiotics commonly found in any veterinary practice are acceptable for use in ocular disease. I feel several are worthy of note; trimethoprim-sulfa, chloramphenicol, and gentamicin, in that order, should be used when retrobulbar abscesses and endophthalmitis are encountered.

Anti-Inflammatory Agents

The injectable corticosteroid of choice is prednisolone. This medication has a half-life of twelve hours. Again, as with the oral medications, if an error in judgment is made, the medication will last about one day. Although dexamethasone and repository steroids have uses in ophthalmology, I believe that they should be used in ocular cases only with the advice of a specialist.

Flunixin meglumine may be administered parenterally at the dosages mentioned above.

Ocular Hypotensive Agents

The injectable hyperosmotic of choice in veterinary medicine is mannitol.[g] Mannitol is convenient and is useful prior to surgery in that oral intake is avoided. It is inexpensive and is effective if fluids are withheld from the patient following use. If mannitol is

---

g. Anpro Pharmaceutical, Arcadia, CA.

given prior to ophthalmic surgery and is immediately followed by crystalline fluids, such as lactated Ringer's solution, the efficacy of the mannitol will be lessened. The dosage for mannitol is the same as for oral glycerin, usually 1 to 2 gm/kg.

Local Anesthetics

Injectable local anesthetic agents such as lidocaine[h] or bupivacaine[i] are used for performing auriculopalpebral nerve blocks in small animals. When intense blepharospasm occurs and the clinician is unable to open the eyelids, 1 to 2 ml of local anesthetic injected directly over the nerve will cause the orbicularis oculi muscle to relax and will greatly facilitate the examination. The site for injection in small animals is just superior to the zygomatic arch between the middle and temporal (posterior) thirds. Mixing local anesthetics with hyaluronidase[j] will allow the anesthetic to spread through surrounding tissues more easily.

TOPICALLY APPLIED OPHTHALMIC DRUGS

Although many topically applied ophthalmic medications come only as liquids and others are available only as ointments, many of the commonly used ophthalmic drugs come as both drops and ointments. In reality, the choice of whether to use drops or ointments should be based on which the client is able to apply more easily to the patient's eye; on species and individual animal tractability differences; on the frequency at which medication is required in relation to the client's ability to administer it; and on the clinician's personal preferences. That the use of ointments does *not* retard the healing of corneal ulcers has been shown experimentally. Ophthalmic ointments tend to be longer lasting but may be slightly more irritating and difficult to apply than suspensions or solutions.

Antimicrobials

The medications gentamicin and gentamicin-betamethasone are widely overprescribed and overused. When gentamicin was a new medication, it was over ninety percent effective against a wide variety of bacteria; now we are lucky if it is fifty percent effective. The reason is because this is the first, and sometimes

---

h. Elkins-Sinn, Inc., Cherry Hill, NJ.
i. Marcaine, Sterling Drug Inc., New York, NY.
j. Wydase, Wyeth Laboratories, Philadelphia, PA.

the only, antibiotic that a veterinary clinician reaches for. I do not even keep this medication in my referral practice because I know that *every* patient that comes in for *any* ocular condition has been on this medication prior to coming to me. I also feel that to use a combination antibiotic-corticosteroid medication is often based on the lack of a specific diagnosis prior to medication being dispensed. Either an antibiotic is necessary or it isn't. Just because a steroidal agent is being used does not mean that an antibiotic is required to "cover" the steroid.

Most conditions seen in a veterinary practice are not infectious when presented; usually we are trying to achieve bacterial prophylaxis. I believe that the best antibiotic for broad-spectrum coverage and efficacy is a combination of neomycin-polymycin B-gramicidin[k] solution or neomycin-polymycin B-bacitracin[l] ointment. If a purulent ocular condition exists, a smear and gram stain can provide guidance in initial selection of an antimicrobial; bacterial culture and sensitivity should be submitted *immediately*. In this way, if the bacteria is resistant to the first antibiotic selected, an antibiotic to which the bacteria is sensitive could be prescribed.

A second antibiotic to keep in the clinic would be tetracycline.[m] This medication is effective in feline chlamydial and mycoplasmal conjunctivitis. More expensive antibiotics may be given via prescription to be filled at a human pharmacy.

Antiviral medications should also be by prescription, as the number of cases of viral infections seen in the general veterinary practice is low, and the expiration date on most medication would be exceeded prior to the medication being used. Trifluridine[n] is probably the most effective antiviral agent for use in feline herpesvirus conjunctivitis, the most common clinical condition for which an antiviral is required. Cases of herpetic keratitis, confirmed by indirect fluorescent antibody testing or virus isolation, should also be treated with trifluridine. If improvement is not noted within two weeks, idoxuridine[o] and vidarabine[p] may also be tried. These medications have been shown to be less effective than trifluridine in treating feline herpetic keratitis.

Antifungal medications are not used often enough in a clinical practice to justify their being stocked in the clinical pharmacy.

---

k. Neosporin ophthalmic solution, Burroughs Wellcome Co., Research Triangle Park, NC.

l. Neosporin ophthalmic ointment, Burroughs Wellcome Co., Research Triangle Park, NC.

m. Terramycin ophthalmic ointment, Pfizer Inc., New York, NY.

n. Viroptic, Burroughs Wellcome Co., Research Triangle Park, NC.

o. Stoxil, Smith Kline & French Laboratories, Philadelphia, PA.

p. Vira-A, Burroughs Wellcome Co., Research Triangle Park, NC.

I believe that any corneal ulcer that does not respond to routine antibiotic treatment should be referred to a specialist for consultation. Antifungal therapy should be initiated only after scraping or culture confirms infection. Although they are not ophthalmic drugs, miconazole[q] or amphotericin B[r] are the drugs of choice in cases of confirmed fungal keratitis. Miconazole is used for topical application just as found in the ampule in which it is shipped. Amphotericin B should be used at a time when no other drugs are being used, as it will form precipitates if it mixes with other drugs; the intravenous preparation is diluted to a concentration of 3 mg percent and applied topically. The drug natamycin[s] may well be the drug of choice in confirmed *Aspergillus* sp. infections but is quite expensive and its use should be reserved for resistant cases as confirmed by sensitivity testing.

Anti-Inflammatory Agents

The commonly used topically applied anti-inflammatory drugs are the corticosteroids. Using steroids in an infected eye is contraindicated. If an antibiotic is indicated, a steroid is rarely necessary in most clinical conditions. If the condition resolves after using antibiotics and the subsequent scarring and vascularization are considered to be nonbeneficial, then corticosteroids may be added to or used in lieu of the antibiotic. To reach for an antibiotic-corticosteroid mixture as the first medication used in any clinical condition would seem to indicate that a specific diagnosis has not been made. As stated above, just the prescription of a topically applied corticosteroid does not indicate the need for an antibiotic to "cover" the steroid.

Two corticosteroid medications provide excellent immunosuppression and retardation of scarring and vascularization *and also impede healing!* Dexamethasone 0.1%[t] or 0.05%[u] is considered to be a mild steroid and 1.0% prednisolone acetate[v] is considered a strong steroid. These are available in generic form and significant savings can be realized by prescribing the generic product. Every practice should have available one of the dexamethasone agents. These have the anti-inflammatory properties to help most cases

---

q. Monistat I.V., Janssen Pharmaceutica, Inc., Piscataway, NJ.

r. Fungizone Intravenous, E. R. Squibb & Sons, Inc., Princeton, NJ.

s. Natacyn, Alcon Laboratories, Inc., Forth Worth, TX.

t. Maxidex ophthalmic suspension, Alcon Laboratories, Inc., Fort Worth, TX.

u. Maxidex ophthalmic ointment, Alcon Laboratories, Inc., Fort Worth, TX.

v. Pred-Forte, Allergan Pharmaceuticals, Inc., Irvine, CA.

seen in a clinical practice and are not likely to cause significant problems if used at an inauspicious time.

Ocular Hypotensive Agents

Glaucoma is commonly seen in a clinical veterinary practice. Unfortunately, it is not often recognized until the eye is buphthalmic. Once the eye is buphthalmic, surgery is often the only treatment that will make the patient comfortable and cosmetic at the same time. For those cases of acute glaucoma that are recognized, I would recommend 1.0% pilocarpine[w] be used topically QID, while awaiting referral to a veterinary ophthalmologist. This medication has several uses in clinical practice. Pilocarpine has been shown to lower the intraocular pressure (IOP) in primary glaucoma, may be used as a prophylactic agent to prolong the time interval of onset of glaucoma between the first eye and the second eye, and may be used orally to stimulate tear production in cases of keratoconjunctivitis sicca (KCS). Cases of secondary glaucoma (i.e., secondary to lens luxation, uveitis, or trauma) will rarely respond to any topically applied medication and will require surgery to alleviate the glaucoma.

Medications such as timolol[x], dipivefrin[y], echothiophate iodide,[z] and demecarium bromide[aa] are expensive to maintain on the hospital shelf, are infrequently used even in a referral practice, and are more easily dispensed by prescription.

Miscellaneous Drugs

Several miscellaneous drugs are of benefit and should be part of every clinical veterinary practice. These include ophthalmic lubricants, artificial tears, collyrium, mydriatics, and topical anesthetics.

Ophthalmic lubricants usually contain white petrolatum and mineral oil[bb] or lanolin[cc] and are useful prior to therapeutic bathing or dipping of dogs and cats. Lubricants are also useful in the occasional patient who develops facial nerve palsy and therefore can no longer blink. The use of a lubricant may help prolong

---

w. Pilocar, CooperVision Ophthalmic Products, San German, Puerto Rico.

x. Timoptic, Merck Sharp & Dohme, West Point, PA.

y. Propine, Allergan Pharmaceuticals, Inc., Irvine, PA.

z. Phospholine iodide, Ayerst Laboratories, New York, NY.

aa. Humorsol, Merck Sharp & Dohme, West Point, PA.

bb. Duolube, Bausch & Lomb, Inc., Pharmaceuticals, Rochester, NY.

cc. Lacrilube-S.O.P., Allergan Pharmaceuticals, Inc., Irvine, NY.

the time interval until exposure keratopathy occurs. In animals with KCS, a lubricant should be used in the eyes before the client goes to work, goes out for a prolonged period of time, and prior to the client going to bed. Animals with lagophthalmos will benefit from use of a lubricant prior to surgery to close the eyelid aperture.

Artificial tears, either polyvinyl alcohol[dd] or hydroxyethylcellulose,[ee] are valuable in the treatment of keratoconjunctivitis sicca (KCS). Tears should be applied in KCS cases as often as possible and at least four to six times a day. Tears may also be applied prior to therapeutic bathing or dipping if lubricant ointments are not available.

Collyrium[ff] is useful for flushing foreign bodies from the corneal surface and for flushing mucus and cellular debris from the conjunctival cul-de-sac in case of KCS. It is easily applied by the client. Using collyrium, excessive fluorescein or rose bengal stain may easily be flushed from eyes.

Every veterinary clinic should have two parasympatholytic mydriatic-cycloplegics, tropicamide[gg] and atropine.[hh] Although any mydriatic should dilate the pupil sufficiently for diagnostic purposes, cycloplegia is important for the relief of the ciliary spasm that occurs with anterior uveitis. Uveitis in any patient should be treated with a mydriatic-cycloplegic as part of the medication regimen. Tropicamide is useful as a mydriatic because a complete fundus and intraocular examination cannot be performed without pupillary dilation; this agent has a faster onset and shorter duration of dilation than atropine and is the drug of choice for clinical ophthalmic examination. Due to its weak cycloplegia, it is often considered a mydriatic. An occasional cat will salivate profusely after the use of tropicamide but that is, in my experience, the exception and not the rule.

Atropine, a cycloplegic and a mydriatic, has a slower onset and longer duration of action than tropicamide, and both ophthalmic ointment and solutions of atropine should be kept in the pharmacy. The use of cycloplegic and/or mydriatic drops in cats may cause profuse salivation and subsequent client noncompliance; I have had clients think that their cats have developed rabies after the use of atropine solutions. I therefore encourage the use of atropine ointments in the cat.

---

dd. Liquifilm, Allergan Pharmaceuticals, Inc., Irvine, CA.

ee. Adsorbotear, Alcon Laboratories, Inc., Fort Worth, TX.

ff. Dacriose, CooperVision Ophthalmic Products, San German, Puerto Rico.

gg. Mydriacyl, Alcon Laboratories, Inc., Fort Worth, TX.

hh. Atropine sulfate 1%, Pharmafair, Inc., Hauppauge, NY.

The topical anesthetic agents of choice for small or large animal practice is proparacaine.[ii,jj] This agent causes less of a burning sensation when topically applied than tetracaine.[kk] Anesthetics are used prior to obtaining a scraping for cytologic examination and flushing the nasolacrimal duct. Topical anesthetic should be applied at the rate of about 1 drop every 30 seconds for 2 to 4 doses. Increasing the frequency will not increase the depth of anesthesia, only the possibility of toxic reactions. In the inflamed eye, anesthesia will not be as pronounced or as long in duration as in the noninflamed eye due to rapid absorption through dilated blood vessels. Anesthesia is enhanced by prior application of one drop of a vasoconstricting agent such as 1:10,000 epinephrine.[ll] Depth of anesthesia may be increased by applying an anesthetic-soaked cotton-tipped applicator to the conjunctival surface for 30 to 60 seconds. Topical anesthetics should be prescribed for a client to use in a patient who is evidencing pain; topical anesthetics are toxic to the corneal epithelium, and repetitive use may lead to significant corneal complications, such as corneal perforation.

ii. Ophthetic, Allergan Pharmaceuticals, Inc., Irvine, CA.
jj. Alcaine, Alcon Laboratories, Inc., Forth Worth, TX.
kk. Tetracaine Hydrochloride 0.5%, Pharmafair, Inc., Hauppauge, NY.
ll. Adrenalin chloride solution, Parke-Davis, Morris Plans, NJ.

Visual Impairment

Arnold Leon

EVALUATION OF VISUAL FUNCTION

Visual History

The history of an animal's visual loss is of great help and importance to the veterinary ophthalmologist. The history may be very characteristic of a certain disease process almost to the extent of being diagnostic.

Onset and duration of visual impairment should be determined by careful questioning of the owners. Lesions causing sudden visual loss include diabetic cataracts, retinal detachment, optic neuritis, complete aqueous or vitreous hemorrhage, CNS or optic nerve trauma, and sudden acquired retinal degeneration (SARD). Gradual-onset blindness may be more suggestive of chronic superficial keratitis, pigmentary keratitis, chronic glaucoma or uveitis, primary or secondary cataracts, or the inherited progressive retinal atrophies. Age at onset can be very helpful, especially with the inherited retinal atrophies, which show distinct breed differences in this respect.

Duration of the visual deficit not only aids diagnosis but also may yield information on prognosis; a visual deficit in a very young animal suggests a congenital lesion such as microphthalmos, congenital cataract, retinal dysplasia, or optic nerve hypoplasia. Chronicity of certain conditions such as retinal detachment or granulomatous uveitis is frequently attended by a poor prognosis, but this is not the case in other conditions such as primary cataract. If the animal does have cataracts, was a visual defect noticed before their development? If so, the cataracts are probably secondary to an inherited retinal degeneration.

Vision during the day and at night should be ascertained from the owners. Day blindness (hemeralopia), sometimes with improved night vision, is suggestive of diseased cone photoreceptors, or it may be a sign of "central" progressive retinal atrophy (CPRA). Night blindness (nyctalopia) usually has a history of the animal bumping into objects in dim light, preferring well-lit rooms, or being "afraid" to remain in dark rooms, and is suggestive of abnormal rod photoreceptor function, as in the generalized progressive retinal atrophies.

Ability to see moving objects should be determined from the history. The peripheral retina is largely responsible for perceiving movement; thus failure to see a thrown ball may suggest diseases such as generalized PRA or peripheral retinal detachment. Ability to see stationary objects should likewise be ascertained; this is a function of the central retina. Thus, an animal's tendency to bump into objects directly in its path or to lose objects that cross from its peripheral to central visual field suggests a lesion of the central retina such as CPRA, central retinal detachment, or a lesion obscuring the visual axis such as nuclear cataracts or persistent hyperplastic primary vitreous (PHPV). If the animal does bump into objects, does it tend to do this on one or both sides?

Abnormal head carriage may be commented on by the owner. For example, on being called, dogs with CPRA may look at their owners with the head turned slightly to one side because they are attempting to use the more functional fundus periphery. Similarly, an animal may hold its head in a lowered position if the superior retina is diseased.

Despite all the useful information that can be obtained by careful questioning of an owner, the clinician should be aware of the pitfalls. A unilaterally blind animal often shows no noticeable evidence of blindness to its owner until the second eye becomes affected. Animals with slowly progressive visual deficits will often adapt extremely well, and the owner may not notice that something is amiss until the animal is placed in a new, unfamiliar environment.

Neurologic History

Visual loss in animals is usually attributable to ocular lesions in most cases, but occasionally a visual defect may result from disease processes of the optic nerves, tracts, or cerebral cortex. Hence, determining if the owner has noticed other neurologic signs such as altered character or reduced alertness can be helpful. Loss of alertness due to cranial nerve or CNS disease can be misinterpreted by owners as a visual defect. The astute clinical ophthalmologist must be a neurologist as well; a history that reveals evidence of other neurologic signs is an indication for a thorough neurologic examination.

General Health

Because ocular disease can be a manifestation of systemic illness, the owner must be questioned about the animal's general health and the presence of other clinical signs, such as weight loss, polydipsia, polyuria, vomiting, or diarrhea; polydipsia accompanying cataracts might indicate diabetes mellitus. The animal's diet may have a bearing on its visual loss; young cats fed dog food may develop taurine-deficiency retinopathy. The owner should also be asked if the animal is on any medication. Atropine drops hinder assessment of pupillary light reflexes; prolonged treatment of colitis using certain lacrimotoxic sulfonamides may be responsible for the development of sight-threatening keratoconjunctivitis sicca (KCS).

Obstacle Course

Photopic

Obstacle courses provide the clinician with one of the best objective assessments of an animal's vision. A simple obstacle course can be quickly constructed by positioning objects such as chairs, tables, rubbish bins, and several boxes at various points and then either calling the animal from the other side of the room (in the case of dogs) or simply observing the animal's movements or encouraging movement (in the case of cats).

The animal's ability to negotiate an obstacle course is first assessed in lighted conditions. If a uniocular visual deficit is suspected, one eye can be covered with a patch and the animal's progress observed. Even blind animals, particularly cats, may negotiate obstacles using other senses (smell and touch/whiskers), albeit with hesitancy. These same animals will bump into objects if hurried through the course by a sudden noise behind them.

Scotopic

The room is then darkened and the animal is run through the obstacle course again. Animals that negotiate the course in photopic conditions but bump into objects in scotopic conditions may have defective rod photoreceptor function, as in the inherited generalized progressive retinal atrophies in dogs.

Menace Response

Animals with normal vision blink when their eyes are menaced by a hand. This test is best performed on each eye in turn by moving the hand towards the eye or upwards into the animal's visual axis so as to minimize air currents that can lead to false positive responses.

In order to elicit a positive menace response, the afferent pathway from retina to visual cortex and the efferent pathway from visual cortex to brain stem and facial nerve (cranial nerve VII) must both be intact. A very bright penlight in a dark room not only tests pupillary light reflexes but also elicits a menace response that causes the animal to blink or shut its eyelids.

The clinician should be aware of the pitfalls of the menace response. Animals not responding to the menace may simply be very passive or they may have CNS disease that is causing decreased alertness or other mental derangement. To overcome these pitfalls, other tests of visual function are useful. One simple method is to hold up a ball, attract the animal's attention to it, and then drop the ball. Most animals will follow the movement of the ball to the floor. Similarly, the animal's ability to follow objects several feet away is another useful test of visual function, particularly with puppies and kittens. These tests must be repeated several times before a negative response is attributed.

Visual field defects are difficult to assess in animals, but an attempt can be made. In a darkened room with one of the animal's eyes covered, watch for corresponding head or eye movements while a penlight is swept across the visual axis in various planes.

Neurologic Examination

Most important in the evaluation of visual function by neuro-ophthalmologic examination is the assessment of the pupillary light reflex (PLR). The afferent pathway involves the retina, optic nerve (II), optic chiasm, rostral optic tract, and pretectum of midbrain to Edinger-Westphal nucleus of the oculomotor nerve (III). The efferent pathway extends from the oculomotor nerve (parasympathetic fibers) to the ciliary ganglion, ciliary body, and iris sphincter muscle.

In a darkened room, a bright light is shone into one eye; normally this causes a rapid and complete pupillary constriction in both eyes. The response of the eye into which the light is being directed is the direct pupillary reflex, whereas the response in the other eye is the indirect or consensual reflex. Both eyes are tested and compared. The responses of the pupils should be equal. The test should be repeated with the penlight directed into the eye at various angles so as to illuminate all areas of the retina (in case of focal retinal disease).

The pupillary light reflex is independent of vision but still provides useful information on the integrity of all components of the afferent and efferent pathways. Blindness with an abnormal PLR localizes the lesion rostral to the lateral geniculate body (LGB). Blindness with a normal PLR reveals the lesion to involve the LGB, optic radiation, or visual cortex.

Electrophysiology

The electroretinogram (ERG) is a recording of the electrical potential generated by the retina across the eyeball in response to a light stimulus. In animals the ERG is usually recorded by means of a corneal contact lens electrode and the responses to a flash of light or repeated flashes (flicker) are displayed on an oscilloscope after amplification.

The normal ERG in domestic animals consists of a number of waves: an initial electronegative *a* wave, followed by an electropositive *b* wave; a later electropositive *c* wave is also seen on DC recordings after a prolonged stimulus.

The clinical ERG is in fact the summation of three separate waveform components classically described by Granit as PI, PII, and PIII. PI corresponds to the *c* wave and is generated by the retinal pigment epithelium in response to a prolonged light stimulus. PII corresponds to the *b* wave and is thought to originate in the inner nuclear layer (bipolar and Müller cells). PIII corresponds to the *a* wave and represents the photoreceptor response. Hence, the ERG can be used to monitor retinal function.

In domestic animals, electroretinography is usually performed under general anesthesia or sedation. The ERG is recorded under light (photopic) and dark (scotopic) conditions, using light stimuli of different intensities, different wavelengths (colored filters), and varying frequencies (flicker-fusion determination) so as to distinguish rod and cone function. Despite the limitations of the procedure, such as lack of standardization of recording equipment and techniques and individual variation in response, electroretinography is not only a useful research tool for investigation of inherited retinal disease but also has several applications in the clinical field:

1. In animals with total cataracts, the PLR is not a reliable indication of retinal health; PLR may be normal with significant retinal disease or abnormal in the presence of a healthy retina if iris atrophy is present. If the fundus cannot be visualized in these animals, the cataracts might be secondary to a retinal degeneration. Before committing the patients to cataract extraction, electroretinography is indicated to ascertain if the retina is functional.

2. Differentiation between optic neuritis and sudden acquired retinal degeneration (SARD) requires electroretinographic examination. In optic neuritis the ERG is unaffected (or minimally affected), whereas in SARD the ERG is extinguished.

3. Early detection of PRA-affected animals is another application. Particularly with certain forms of PRA, such as rod-cone dysplasia in the Irish Setter, electroretinographic diagnosis may

be made at several weeks of age, before there is ophthalmoscopic evidence of the disease.

The visual evoked cortical potential (VEP) is a recording of the electrical activity of the brain elicited by a visual stimulus. The VEP is recorded using scalp electrodes placed at certain positions over the cortex in a manner similar to an electroencephalogram (EEG) recording. The stimulus used may be a flash of light or the presentation of a pattern on a screen or TV monitor.

Because of the background noise and because the electrical signals generated are so small, the stimulus is repeated many times and VEP is recorded as an averaged response, usually on an oscilloscope. In animals the VEP is usually recorded with the subject anesthetized (depending on species), although certain anesthetic agents can suppress the response. A characteristic waveform is produced that varies greatly depending on the position of the recording electrodes on the scalp, the type of stimulus used, and the individual. In most cases the VEP waveform comprises a series of electropositive peaks and electronegative troughs.

The VEP is currently a research tool, but it may have evolving clinical applications involving the assessment of diseases of the optic nerve and the central visual system.

CONGENITAL DISEASE ASSOCIATED WITH VISUAL IMPAIRMENT

Conditions Involving the Globe as a Whole

Anophthalmos, Microphthalmos, and Nanophthalmos

Anophthalmos is complete absence of the globe resulting from failure in development of the optic vesicle from the cerebral vesicle. True anophthalmos is rare in all species. Apparent or clinical anophthalmos represents most cases seen in practice in which the eye is apparently absent, but some ocular tissue can be detected histologically.

Microphthalmos is the presence of an abnormal, small globe resulting from retarded or aberrant development of the optic vesicle. Other cystic structures may be present. It is usually associated with multiple congenital ocular anomalies including colobomata, retinal nonattachment, cataracts, and persistent pupillary membranes with consequent visual impairment. Nanophthalmos is uncomplicated microphthalmos, the presence of a small but otherwise normal globe. These conditions may occur unilaterally or bilaterally. Microphthalmos and nanophthalmos are relatively common in the dog.

ETIOLOGIES

Vitamin A deficiency

Hereditary causes are common in several canine breeds, including the Collie breeds, Doberman Pinscher, Australian Shepherd Dog, and Miniature Schnauzer.

Toxic causes (teratogenic agents) of anophthalmos and/or microphthalmos include griseofulvin in the cat.

Idiopathic and/or spontaneous causes of microphthalmos account for many cases seen in practice.

CLINICAL FINDINGS

Anophthalmic and grossly microphthalmic eyes should present no problems in recognition. Difficulties, however, do arise with very mild cases of microphthalmos or nanophthalmos in which the globe is only slightly reduced in size. In such cases the following features may be of help in comparing a unilaterally affected eye with its normal companion eye:

The affected eye may show slight enophthalmos. Compare the two eyes by looking down vertically from above the animal's head.

The third eyelid may be slightly more prominent on the affected side.

The affected globe may show more exposed sclera and there may be microcornea with an abnormal limbus.

Other ocular defects may be present, including cataract, retinal detachment, and coloboma.

DIFFERENTIAL DIAGNOSIS

In phthisis bulbi, the globe is grossly shrunken as a result of chronic glaucoma, inflammation, or trauma destroying the ciliary body. Microphthalmos is seen in young animals, and there is no history or other evidence of antecedent ocular disease or trauma. Microphthalmic eyes do not tend to have the shrunken, wrinkled appearance of phthisical globes.

PROGNOSIS AND TREATMENT

Microphthalmos cannot be treated, and the prognosis for the animal depends on the individual case: the severity of the lesion and degree of visual impairment, whether the lesion is unilateral or bilateral, and the use for which the animal is required. In young companion animals with bilateral severe disease, euthanasia may be the preferred alternative. Less severe cases may lead a reasonable life provided other ocular anomalies (cataracts) do not progress, but their use for future breeding should be avoided, particularly in those breeds in which the condition is known to be hereditary. Chronic conjunctivitis associated with tear retention by an enlarged lacrimal lake may be managed with daily irrigation and topical antibiotics or, in severe cases, by enucleation.

Congenital Glaucoma

Goniodysgenesis or abnormal differentiation of the iridocorneal angle may result in an animal born with an enlarged globe due to obstructed drainage of aqueous humor. The more severe condition of anterior segment dysgenesis may also cause congenital glaucoma.

INCIDENCE

Rare, sporadic condition
Inherited condition in the Doberman Pinscher

CLINICAL FINDINGS

Unilateral or bilateral enlarged globe; buphthalmos occurs more readily and markedly in young animals.
Eye is blind with a raised intraocular pressure
Corneal opacities, pupils fixed and dilated, tapetal fundus hyperreflectivity, attenuated retinal blood vessels, cupping of the optic disc, and optic atrophy.

TREATMENT

Surgical alternatives for cosmesis are described in this chapter.

Congenital Corneal Opacification

Ophthalmia Neonatorum

This is an infectious keratoconjunctivitis of the neonatal animal seen in both dogs and cats and most commonly in kittens up to four weeks old.

CLINICAL FINDINGS

Unilateral or bilateral swollen eyelids due to accumulation of pus within a closed conjunctival sac
Purulent exudate may appear at the medial canthus
If due to herpes virus infection, in kittens other signs may be evident, such as rhinitis and bronchopneumonia; other kittens in the litter may be similarly affected.

The following possible sequelae all cause visual impairment due to corneal opacification:

Corneal ulceration and/or perforation and resultant corneal scars and anterior synechiae

Symblepharon (adhesions of conjunctiva to cornea or itself) is a common sequel.
Panophthalmitis, phthisis bulbi

Therapy of this condition is described in Chapter 5.

Persistent Pupillary Membranes (PPM)

Persistent pupillary membranes are a cause of congenital corneal opacity due to remnants of the embryonic pupillary membrane adhering to the posterior corneal surface. The condition is inherited in the Basenji probably genetic in the Collie, and frequently occurs spontaneously in all breeds. Corneal opacification is rarely so extensive as to affect vision; rarely corneas with extensive PPM will experience endothelial decompensation with resultant edema.

CLINICAL FINDINGS

A focal white corneal opacity is usually seen with one or more adherent strands of tissue running back to join the midportion (collarette) of the iris. These strands may be very fine and difficult to detect without suitable means of magnification. Distinguishing PPMs from posterior synechiae is based on origin, the latter arising from the pupillary margin.

The corneal lesion associated with PPMs may resemble a scar resulting from a perforating injury. Differentiate as follows:

PPM is congenital without history of ocular trauma
With a PPM the corneal epithelium is intact and not roughened and the corneal opacity deep with a normal overlying stroma.
The eye is quiescent and comfortable.
Other small PPM tags may sometimes be seen on the iris collarette.

Anterior Segment Dysgenesis

This is a developmental anomaly of ocular neuroectodermal tissues probably caused by a defect of the optic cup. This defect results in multiple ocular malformations including microphthalmos, retinal dysplasia, and abnormalities of the iris and ciliary body epithelium with associated abnormal development of the cornea, anterior chamber, anterior uvea, lens (aphakia), and vitreous. The syndrome may be inherited as a recessive trait in the Doberman Pinscher and St. Bernard breeds with several affected pups in a litter.

INCIDENCE

Sporadically recorded in the dog and cat

CLINICAL FINDINGS

Blindness due to bilateral multiple ocular anomalies

Microphthalmos of varying degrees

Congenital glaucoma may be present.

Corneal opacification obscures examination of the interior of the eye.

Several animals in the litter may be affected.

DIAGNOSIS

Congenital condition

Findings of ophthalmic examination

Breed incidence

DIFFERENTIAL DIAGNOSIS

Other diseases combining microphthalmos with multiple congenital ocular anomalies; in these conditions the cornea is usually opaque and permits visualization of other ocular structures.

Ophthalmia neonatorum resulting in corneal scarring. The corneal surface is irregular and there may be evidence of perforation. Microphthalmos is absent.

PROGNOSIS AND TREATMENT

Treatment is impossible. Because of the several bilateral visual defect, such animals should be destroyed.

Congenital Lens Opacification

Congenital Cataracts

Congenital cataracts may be associated with a normal-sized and normal-shaped lens, or they may be associated with abnormal lens morphology.

Abnormal Lens Shape

Microphakia/Spherophakia

In this condition the lens is smaller than normal and may be round or bean-shaped (Figure 4–1). It may be accompanied by multiple congenital ocular anomalies in the Doberman Pinscher, St. Bernard, and Beagle dogs and is commonly encountered in Miniature Schnauzers associated with congenital cataracts.

APPEARANCE

Unilateral or bilateral

Elongated ciliary processes are seen surrounding the small, misshapen lens, the borders of which are fully visible when the pupils are dilated.

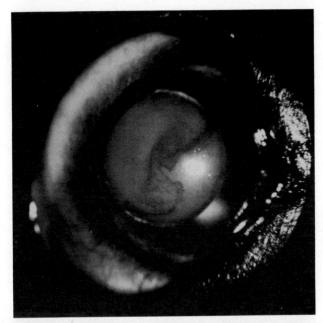

FIGURE 4-1. Microphakia and spherophakia in the right eye of a young hound. Note the pigment on the anterior lens capsule. The condition was bilateral; intracapsular lens removal and anterior vitrectomy was successful.

The lens may be cataractous with associated visual impairment. Nystagmus is sometimes seen.

Posterior Lenticonus and Lentiglobus

This is a congenital malformation of the lens wherein the posterior surface exhibits an axial conical protrusion into the vitreous body; lentiglobus is more severe than lenticonus. It occurs sporadically in several species including the dog and may also be seen as part of several syndromes with multiple congenital ocular anomalies.

APPEARANCE

Usually unilateral

Protrusion of the posterior lens into the vitreous may require slitlamp biomicroscopy for detection. Very severe cases are obvious on direct visualization (Figure 4-2).

The lens may be cataractous with associated visual deficit.

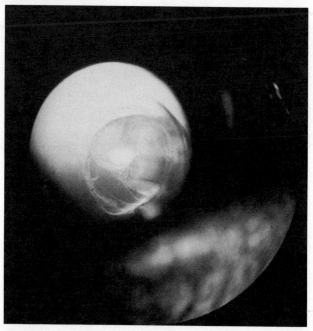

FIGURE 4-2. Unilateral posterior lenticonus in the right eye of a Golden Retriever puppy demonstrating the typical "oil droplet" cataract associated with this condition.

Lens Coloboma

This is an uncommon lesion in which part of the lens is absent; usually inferiorly, resulting in a flattened equatorial contour at 6 o'clock. It is invariably accompanied by colobomata of the adjacent ciliary body and zonular fibers and may be part of a syndrome with multiple congenital ocular anomalies.

APPEARANCE

Mild cases are apparent as a notch or notches on the lens equator, usually at six o'clock.

Severe colobomata may be evident in which much of the lens has apparently failed to develop.

Adjacent cortical cataracts are commonly seen, which tend to be very slowly progressive.

Normal Lens Shape

Persistent Pupillary Membranes

Remnants of the pupillary membrane may adhere to the anterior lens capsule and cause varying degrees of congenital lens opacification (Figure 4–3). The lesions are nonprogressive and may be part of a syndrome of multiple congenital ocular anomalies.

APPEARANCE

Very mild cases are commonly seen in dogs in which small brown pigmented foci (pigmented capsular flecks) are aggregated on the central anterior lens capsule and do not interfere with vision (Figure 4–4).

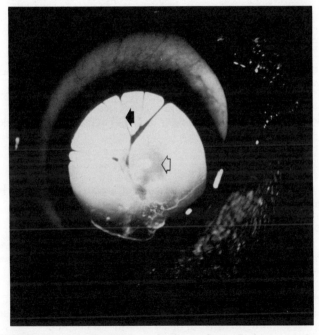

FIGURE 4–3. Anterior capsular and subcapsular cortical cataracts (*open arrow*) associated with persistent pupillary membranes (*solid arrow*) in the right eye of a young American Cocker Spaniel. The pupil has been dilated pharmacologically.

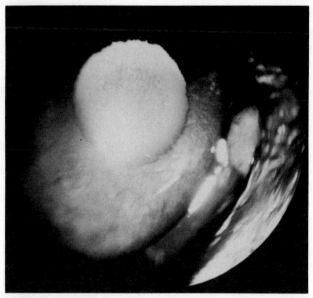

FIGURE 4-4. Pigmented capsular flecks in the right eye of a young Dachshund.

Severe cases are rare but may cause extensive anterior capsular and subcapsular cataracts with nystagmus and visual impairment.

PROGNOSIS AND TREATMENT

These opacities are nonprogressive. Cataract surgery may be considered in severe cases.

Congenital Nuclear and Cortical Cataracts

This condition most commonly involves the nucleus of the lens and represents insults that have affected the primary lens fibers during the earliest stage of lens development.

ETIOLOGY

Some cases are hereditary; inherited congenital or early-onset cataracts are discussed in detail later in this chapter.

Some cases are idiopathic.

Any noxious influence (trauma, nutritional deficiency, toxic agents, infection, radiation) acting at the time of development of the primary lens fibers early in gestation may result in nuclear cataracts. The condition may be part of a syndrome of multiple congenital ocular anomalies, such as microphthalmos and posterior lenticonus in the Miniature Schnauzer and Cavalier King Charles Spaniel.

APPEARANCE

Appearance will vary from nuclear flecks (seen most commonly in German Shepherds) to diffuse nuclear opacity to a spherical perinuclear opacity seen at the center of the lens to total opacification.

Lens cortex is frequently clear (healthy lens fibers having been laid down around the cataractous nucleus), but occasionally some cortical extensions may be seen.

Nystagmus may be present.

PROGNOSIS AND TREATMENT

Most nuclear cataracts are nonprogressive and indeed may appear to decrease in size as healthy cortical fibers are laid down around them. Topical mydriatics may be utilized to enhance peripheral vision if nuclear cataracts are dense. Total congenital cataracts must be operated early in life to allow light and form stimulation of the central visual centers during their transient period of plasticity. A wandering nystagmus in patients with congenital cataracts is suggestive of failure of this stimulus to occur and warrants a guarded visual prognosis.

Persistent Hyaloid Artery

In this condition the hyaloid artery (a persistent remnant of the vascular supply to the embryonic lens) is present between the optic disc and the axial posterior lens surface. It rarely causes visual impairment except when associated with a posterior capsular cataract. It occurs spontaneously in all species.

CLINICAL FINDINGS

Unilateral or bilateral

A central focal posterior capsular cataract (Mittendorf's dot) (Figure 4–5) may be evident, behind which a hyaloid artery (sometimes containing blood) may be seen stretching back into the vitreous body toward its origin at the optic disk. Occasionally the hyaloid vessel arises from an anomalous superficial retinal vessel.

Rarely the persistent hyaloid artery is accompanied by an extensive posterior capsular and subcapsular cataract that can impede vision.

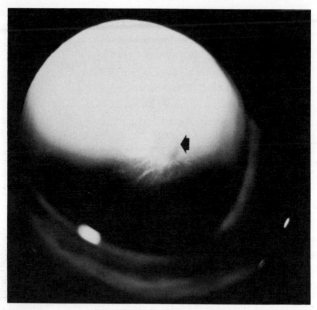

FIGURE 4-5. Persistent anterior hyaloid (Mittendorf's dot) (*arrow*) in an Irish Setter.

PROGNOSIS AND TREATMENT

Posterior capsular cataracts associated with a persistent hyaloid artery tend to be nonprogressive. Unilateral cases require no treatment. Bilateral cases with small posterior capsular cataracts also do not require treatment. Bilateral cases with extensive posterior capsular cataracts are very rare. Medical treatment involves instillation of mydriatic drops (1% atropine approximately every 3 days) to dilate the pupils and extend the animal's visual field. Surgical treatment of severe cases by intracapsular lens extraction and anterior vitrectomy is possible but complicated by the presence of the hyaloid artery, which may require cautery.

Persistent Hyperplastic Primary Vitreous (PHPV)/ Persistent Hyperplastic Tunica Vasculosa Lentis (PHTVL)

PHPV/PHTVL is an uncommon congenital ocular anomaly caused by a failure in regression of the normally transient hyaloid-tunica vasculosa lentis system (the vascular supply that envelops the developing lens). Accompanying fibroplasia results in a plaque of fibrovascular tissue on the posterior surface of the lens.

ETIOLOGY

Sporadic cases are probably caused by some noxious influence acting on the embryonic eye at midgestation or soon thereafter.

In the dog, PHPV has been recorded as an hereditary condition in the Doberman Pinscher and Staffordshire Bull Terrier breeds; it is thought to be inherited as an autosomal dominant gene with incomplete penetrance.

CLINICAL FINDINGS

Sporadic Cases. Sporadic cases can be either unilateral or bilateral.

Leukocoria (white pupil)

Mydriasis reveals a white fibrous plaque containing a network of blood vessels on the posterior aspect of the lens (Figure 4–6). Pigment may also be present.

The plaque of tissue usually has an irregular border, and the peripheral area of the lens is not involved.

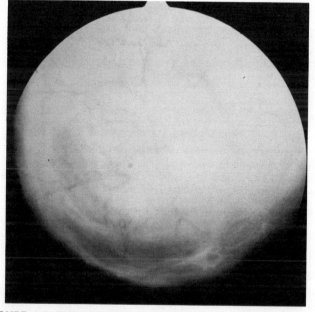

FIGURE 4–6. PHPV/PHTVL of the right eye in a young Doberman Pinscher. The fellow eye was also affected. There is a diffuse posterior capsular opacity axially with an associated vascular network.

Hereditary Cases. Mild hereditary cases have only multiple brown pigment foci scattered over the posterior lens capsule, not affecting vision, and occur unilaterally or bilaterally.

Severe cases are invariably bilateral.

The retrolental plaque of tissue usually contains multiple brown pigment foci and a vascular network.

Other lens anomalies may be present, such as microphakia, colobomata, posterior lenticonus, cataract, or intralenticular hemorrhage.

Other animals in the litter are frequently affected.

Both sporadic and hereditary cases of PHPV may exhibit persistent capsulopupillary vessels (sometimes containing blood) that course from the anterior surface of the iris, loop over the rim of the pupil, and run over the equator of the lens back to the retrolental plaque. These vessels may be associated with lens and ciliary body colobomata.

Vision in bilateral severe cases is considerably reduced, yet these dogs often cope very well by utilizing the clear lens periphery. Affected Dobermans, however, tend to show fear or aggressive behavior as a result of their visual deficit and are also more likely to develop total cataracts.

DIAGNOSIS

Congenital condition
Characteristic ophthalmic appearance
Possible breed incidence

DIFFERENTIAL DIAGNOSIS

Other causes of leukocoria include:

Cataracts
Total retinal detachment or nonattachment
Posterior segment tumor
Organized intraocular hemorrhage
Endophthalmitis or vitreous abscess

PHPV is differentiated from all these conditions in that it is congenital, the opacity is situated on the posterior lens capsule and is vascularized, vision is present, pupillary light reflexes are normal, and the eye is not inflamed.

PROGNOSIS

Unilateral cases require no treatment. Bilateral cases may also not need treatment if vision is not greatly impaired. Severe bilateral cases can be treated medically or surgically, but euthanasia may be preferable if the animal is very young and has already developed intralenticular hemorrhage or total cataracts. Doberman Pinschers or Staffordshire Bull Terriers with PHPV should not be used for breeding, even if only mildly affected.

TREATMENT

Medical: topical application of 1% atropine drops every 3 to 4 days will maintain mydriasis and extend the dog's visual field if total cataracts are not present.

Surgical: if total cataracts are present, surgical extraction is possible but frequently complicated. An intracapsular extraction with anterior vitrectomy has achieved the best results.

Congenital Vitreous Opacification

Congenital vitreous opacification is uncommon and usually due to hemorrhage associated with congenital retinal abnormalities. In these conditions hemorrhage results from tearing of blood vessels in a detached retina or from retinal neovascularization.

ETIOLOGY

Collie eye anomaly (CEA) in Collie breeds

Total retinal dysplasia or retinal nonattachment (Labrador Retriever, Sealyham Terrier, Bedlington Terrier and, occasionally, the English Springer Spaniel)

Multiple congenital ocular anomalies with retinal detachment (Australian Shepherd Dog)

Degenerating hyaloid artery (uncommon in dog and cat)

Preretinal arteriolar loops and other vascular malformations may predispose the eye to intraocular hemorrhage.

CLINICAL FINDINGS

Hemorrhage within the vitreous body, sufficient to impair vision, is easily diagnosed by a red reflex and presence of blood behind the lens as seen with a penlight or ophthalmoscope. Hyphema may also be seen as blood passes forward into the anterior segment of the eye.

DIAGNOSIS

Examination of the fellow eye is essential to detect evidence of CEA, retinal dysplasia and multiple congenital ocular anomalies. Note also the breed incidence of these conditions.

DIFFERENTIAL DIAGNOSIS

Intralenticular hemorrhage in severe cases of PHPV. The hemorrhage in PHPV is within the retrolental plaque of tissue and sometimes also within the lens. The retrolental plaque may be visualized behind the hemorrhage. Breed incidence of PHPV should be considered.

Hyphema may resemble vitreous hemorrhage; indeed, the two conditions have some common causes including congenital retinal and posterior segment anomalies (CEA with retinal detachment, trauma, foreign body penetration, severe uveitis, glaucoma, neoplasia, and blood clotting disorders).

Intravitreal hemorrhage not associated with congenital conditions such as acquired retinal detachment, coagulopathies, and ocular trauma

PROGNOSIS

Congenital intravitreal hemorrhage is serious because it usually indicates a severe disorder of the posterior segment (such as CEA with retinal detachment). This is especially true if the blood remains unclotted, implying continued bleeding. The retina is frequently detached in these animals, and the vitreous may be abnormal. The prognosis for return of vision is hopeless. If the hemorrhage does clear, the vitreous may undergo degenerative changes such as syneresis (liquefaction) and, less commonly, synchisis scintillans, with subsequent retinal detachment if this is not already present. Hemorrhage may also recur with possible sequelae of glaucoma, anterior uveitis, or phthisis bulbi.

Those cases in which intravitreal hemorrhage is due to a degenerating hyaloid artery or preretinal vascular loop may not be so serious, the blood clotting and being resorbed over a period of weeks to months. Even these cases may develop traction retinal detachments.

TREATMENT

Treatment of congenital intravitreal hemorrhage is of no avail. Toxic blood products may cause an anterior uveitis, which can be treated with topical atropine and corticosteroids.

Retina and Optic Nerve

Retinal Dysplasia (RD)

Hereditary/Spontaneous Retinal Dysplasia in the Dog; Multifocal Retinal Dysplasia (Retinal Folds)

This is a congenital ocular anomaly caused by abnormal differentiation of the various retinal layers. Histopathology reveals retinal folds and rosettes due to photoreceptor disorientation.

ETIOLOGY

In all cases of hereditary retinal dysplasia in which the mode of inheritance is known, the disease is inherited as an autosomal recessive trait. An exception may be in some cases the Labrador Retriever breed.

BREED INCIDENCE

Labrador Retriever, American Cocker Spaniel, English Springer Spaniel, Beagle, Rottweiler, Cavalier King Charles Spaniel, Golden Retriever, and possibly Puli.

CLINICAL FINDINGS

In multifocal RD, there are bilateral multiple linear, vermiform, oval, or Y-shaped streaks in the fundus. These folds are dark gray against the background of the tapetal fundus (Figure 4-7,*A*) and white against the non-tapetal fundus (Figure 4-7,*B*).

The folds may occupy certain sites. Folds around the superior retinal blood vessels dorsal to the optic disk are typical of RD in the English Springer Spaniel and Labrador Retriever.

Vision is unaffected.

Lesions remain static (exception: affected English Springer Spaniels may also show multiple areas of tapetal hyperreflectivity and pigmentation, resembling chorioretinitis lesions, as part of multifocal RD (Figure 4-8). These lesions sometimes show slight progression by extension. If these chorioretinitis-like lesions are very extensive, there will be large scotomata and a visual deficit must be present.)

Retinal folds may sometimes be seen in puppies of any breed. Often these folds will disappear as the animal matures and the globe grows.

DIAGNOSIS

Breed incidence
Ophthalmoscopic appearance

DIFFERENTIAL DIAGNOSIS

Retinal folds adjacent to inflammatory lesions or focal flat or bullous retinal detachments. A major diagnostic challenge occurs in the English Springer Spaniel with RD in which both chorioretinitis-like lesions and bullous retinal detachments may be seen. The young age of the dog and the presence of RD lesions in other puppies in the litter should help to differentiate between hereditary RD and acquired postinflammatory lesions in this breed. In isolated older dogs, the ophthalmologist faces a dilemma and must attempt to identify the more typical RD folds elsewhere in the fundus in order to make a diagnosis.

PROGNOSIS

Vision in animals affected with multifocal RD is good (with the possible exception of some English Springer Spaniels) and

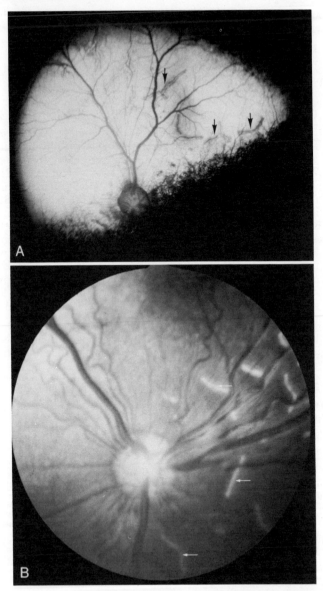

FIGURE 4-7. Retinal folds (*arrows*) in a seven-month-old American Cocker Spaniel (*A*) and a Collie pup (*B*). Figure *A* courtesy of Dr. Alan MacMillan.

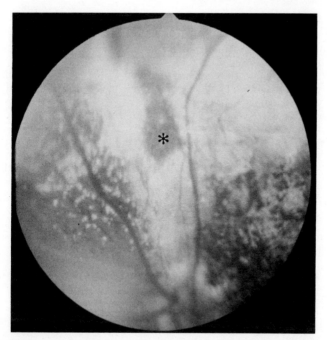

FIGURE 4–8. Extensive RD with "chorioretinitis-like" pigmentary change (∘) in the tapetum of a two-year-old English Springer Spaniel.

is likely to remain so. Affected animals and their parents and offspring should not be used for breeding because, even though vision is unaffected, the more severe manifestation of RD—retinal detachment and blindness—may yet occur in these breeds.

Total Retinal Dysplasia

This is the second, less common hereditary form of RD seen in the dog. It is a congenital abnormality in which the poorly differentiated retina is detached (nonattached). The secondary vitreous may also be absent.

ETIOLOGY

Autosomal recessive trait

BREED INCIDENCE

Sealyham Terrier, Bedlington Terrier, Labrador Retriever, Australian Shepherd Dog. English Springer Spaniels may occasionally present with bilateral retinal detachment.

CLINICAL FINDINGS

Total blindness due to bilateral involvement

Pupils dilated or semidilated with absent or very sluggish pupillary light reflexes

With a penlight, the detached retina is visible lying against the posterior surface of the lens, causing leukocoria (white pupil).

Nystagmus may be present.

Labrador Retrievers may also show cataracts and skeletal abnormalities.

Australian Shepherd Dogs may also exhibit central corneal opacities, heterochromic and hypoplastic irides, abnormal pupil shape and size (dyscoria), cataracts, and staphylomata in the posterior segment (a thinning or outpouching of the sclera, which is lined by uveal tissue).

DIAGNOSIS

Breed incidence
Ophthalmic findings

DIFFERENTIAL DIAGNOSIS

Other causes of leukocoria:

Cataracts. Opacity is within the lens, not posterior to it.

PHPV. Vision is present and pupillary light reflexes are usually normal.

Posterior segment neoplasia occurs in older dogs.

Endophthalmitis. Rarely bilateral. Eye is inflamed and painful.

Organized intraocular hemorrhage. Not congenital; history or evidence of trauma to the globe

Retinal detachment due to other causes. No breed incidence; older dogs (except Collie breeds with CEA); may be accompanied by systemic illness.

PROGNOSIS AND TREATMENT

Therapy is not effective; blindness is permanent and affected eyes may develop rubeosis iridis with repeated bouts of intraocular hemorrhage with the possible sequelae of neovascular glaucoma, anterior uveitis, and phthisis bulbi. Euthanasia of affected puppies is preferable.

Affected animals, their parents, and their offspring should not be used for breeding.

Noninherited Retinal Dysplasia

Abnormal retinal differentiation with formation of retinal folds and rosettes occurs spontaneously in many species, including dogs and cats.

ETIOLOGY

Maternal infections—canine herpes virus and adenovirus; feline panleukopenia and leukemia virus
Intrauterine trauma
Irradiation
Vitamin A deficiency
Certain antiviral drugs
Idiopathic

CLINICAL FINDINGS

Mild cases show multiple retinal folds, visible ophthalmoscopically as linear and vermiform streaks across the fundus. Vision is unaffected.
Severe cases show detached, dysplastic retinas with consequent visual impairment.
Other signs of ocular inflammation may be present (e.g., cataracts, anterior uveitis, and synechiae), particularly if infectious agents are involved.

TREATMENT

Treatment of retinal dysplasia is not effective. Any accompanying ocular inflammation may be treated with corticosteroids and atropine.

Retinal Detachment

Collie Eye Anomaly (CEA)

Collie eye anomaly is a congenital inherited ocular anomaly wherein the principal lesions are choroidal hypoplasia and colobomata of the posterior pole of the eye.

ETIOLOGY

Autosomal recessive trait

BREED INCIDENCE

Rough Collie, Smooth Collie, Shetland Sheepdog, and Border Collie. Incidence is highest in the rough and smooth Collie, with up to ninety percent of animals affected.

CLINICAL FINDINGS

A wide range of severities of CEA may be observed. Most have little or no effect on vision, but the few severely affected dogs (with retinal detachment and/or intraocular hemorrhage) are blind or have grossly defective sight.

Bilateral, but not necessarily symmetrical lesions

Choroidal hypoplasia is seen in most CEA cases and is visible as a focal lesion just lateral or slightly dorsolateral to the optic disk, usually at the tapetal-nontapetal junction. The focal lesion consists of an irregular to oval area lacking pigment and tapetum and exposing the white sclera, overlying which can be seen abnormal choroidal blood vessels. Choroidal vessels may be absent, but are more usually abnormally broad and form bizarre patterns (Figure 4–9,A). Choroidal hypoplasia is diagnostic of CEA. Vision in dogs with only choroidal hypoplasia is normal.

Colobomata are the second most common lesion in CEA (twenty to thirty percent of affected dogs). A coloboma is seen ophthalmoscopically as a gray-colored pit either in the optic disk or in the adjacent peripapillary region. Small colobomata may be difficult to detect because of their size and because they may resemble the physiologic pit in the center of the disk. Larger colobomata are obvious as deep excavations with retinal blood vessels dipping over their rim and disappearing into the depths (Figure 4–9,B). Deep colobomata often involve sclera, and large colobomata of the papilla can involve the whole optic disk. The bottom of these pits may be brought into focus by using negative lenses in the direct ophthalmoscope. Colobomata do not cause defective vision unless they are very extensive optic disk colobomata. A coloboma in the absence of choroidal hypoplasia is somewhat controversially regarded by some authorities as also being diagnostic of CEA.

Retinal detachments in CEA may be partial (flat or bullous) or complete with or without peripheral disinsertion and tearing of the retina (Figure 4–9,C). They occur usually within the first few months of life and rarely develop after one year of age. Vision is affected, depending on the extent of the detachment.

Intraocular hemorrhage may prevent visualization of the fundus in CEA. Both vitreous hemorrhage and hyphema may be present. Hemorrhage is usually, but not always, associated with retinal detachment. The affected eye is often blind.

DIFFERENTIAL DIAGNOSIS

Total retinal dysplasia is the other most common cause of congenital retinal detachment with or without intraocular hemorrhage. RD does not occur in the Collie breeds. Examination of the fellow eye reveals lesions typical of CEA in the Collie breeds.

PROGNOSIS AND TREATMENT

Treatment of CEA is not required in most cases in which vision is unaffected. Vision will not deteriorate. While early cases of partial retinal detachment in Collies have been successfully treated surgically by specialists, eyes with complete retinal detachment and/or intraocular hemorrhage are usually irreparably blind and treatment is not feasible. However, complications of hemorrhage, such as anterior uveitis, may be treated symptomatically (mydriatics and corticosteroids topically). Rubeosis iridis may cause hyphema and/or neovascular glaucoma later in life.

Affected animals (even mild cases), their parents, and their progeny should not be used for breeding.

Posterior Segment Colobomata

A *coloboma* is a congenital tissue defect manifested by a pit, hole, fissure, or notch in any ocular tissue. Posterior segment colobomata may affect retina, choroid, sclera, and/or optic disk. Optic disk colobomata are the most common. Posterior segment colobomata may be accompanied by colobomata of the iris and eyelid. All species are affected.

ETIOLOGY

So-called typical colobomata are seen in the six o'clock meridian of the eye and represent a failure of fusion of the fetal fissure in the midline. Optic disk colobomata in the Collie breeds are part of CEA and inherited as an autosomal recessive trait. Hereditary optic disk colobomata have also been recorded in Basenji dogs. Other causes include retinal pigment epithelial defects and color dilution factors.

In cats typical colobomata of the choroid and iris have been reported with dominant inheritance.

CLINICAL FINDINGS

Very extensive optic disk colobomata may cause blindness (rare in dogs). Smaller colobomata may cause some visual impairment but frequently have minimal or no effect on vision. Retinal and choroidal colobomata have no apparent effect on the animal's vision, although blind spots probably exist.

Unilateral or bilateral in dogs

Pits or holes of variable size are visible in the optic disk.

Blood vessels dip over the rim of the coloboma and disappear into its depths. The bottom of the defect may be brought into focus using negative lenses in the direct ophthalmoscope (often −20 to −30 diopters).

DIFFERENTIAL DIAGNOSIS

Peripapillary chorioretinitis has a hyperreflective area, often with a pigmented border, adjacent to the optic disk. Vessels running over the area of chorioretinitis are frequently attenuated, but do not dip over the edge of the lesion.

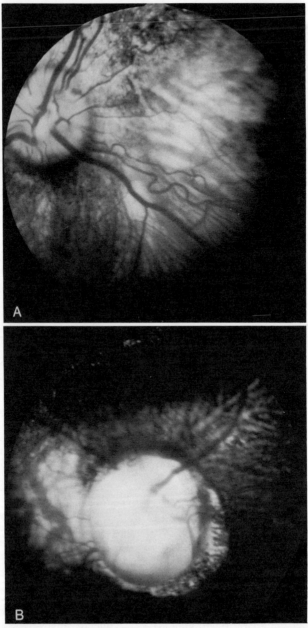

FIGURE 4-9. *See legend on opposite page.*

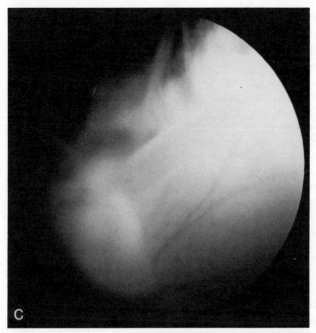

FIGURE 4–9. Collie eye anomaly. *A*, Choroidal hypoplasia temporal to the optic disk in the left eye of a one-year-old sable Collie. The anomalous choroidal vasculature and underlying sclera are readily visible. *B*, Optic disk coloboma in the right eye of a three-year-old tricolor Collie. Temporally, choroidal hypoplasia can be seen; a nasal conus (crescent-shaped area of absence of retinal pigmented epithelium and choroid) is also present. The entire nerve head is depressed; note the retinal vessels disappearing over the edge of the defect. *C*, Total retinal detachment, right eye, in a young sable Collie.

Normal hyperreflective arc dorsal to the optic disk in some dogs (inaccurately referred to as *conus*, Figure 4–9,*B*).

PROGNOSIS AND TREATMENT

No treatment is possible. Colobomata of the posterior segment are not progressive. In dogs vision is rarely affected except with very severe optic disk colobomata. Even if vision in one eye is poor, the other eye usually has good sight.

Optic Nerve Hypoplasia and Aplasia

Optic Nerve Aplasia

This refers to a total failure in development of the optic nerve. It occurs sporadically in any animal but is very rare.

CLINICAL FINDINGS

The eye is blind and may be microphthalmic.

Ophthalmoscopy reveals absence of retinal blood vessels and no visible optic disk, although a small depression may be seen at the posterior pole of the eye.

Optic Nerve Hypoplasia

This refers to abnormal differentiation of the ganglion cell and nerve fiber layers of the retina, resulting in a hypoplastic optic nerve and optic chiasm. It is an uncommon condition of unknown etiology, although genetic tendencies have been incriminated in several breeds.

CLINICAL FINDINGS

Often unilateral and therefore unnoticed by owners

Bilateral cases tend to be blind.

May accompany microphthalmos

The direct pupillary light reflex is sluggish or absent. Consensual reflex is normal if only one optic nerve is hypoplastic.

Optic disk is small, sometimes with a darkly pigmented border and a depressed center.

Retinal blood vessels are normal (Figure 4–10).

Optic nerve hypoplasia is difficult to diagnose ophthalmoscopically in the cat because of the normally small, dark, and depressed nature of the optic disk in this species.

DIFFERENTIAL DIAGNOSIS

Micropapilla is a normal variant in which the optic disk is small (most frequently seen in Belgian Sheepdogs), but the optic nerve is normal. Vision and pupillary light reflexes are normal.

Optic atrophy usually has a history of antecedent ocular disease or trauma. There may be ophthalmoscopic evidence of peripapillary inflammatory lesions.

TREATMENT

None is available.

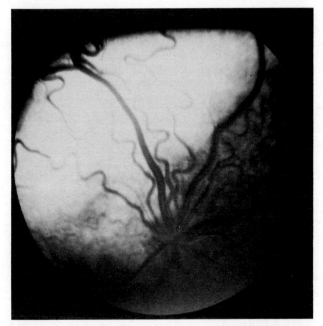

FIGURE 4-10. Optic disk hypoplasia in an eight-week-old Beagle pup.

Central Nervous System

Hydrocephalus

Hydrocephalus results in dilation of the lateral ventricles and interferes with the optic radiation in the lateral walls of these ventricles.

CLINICAL FINDINGS

Bilateral blindness
Bilateral fixed, dilated pupils
Ventrolateral strabismus
Nystagmus is often present.
Papilledema or optic atrophy may be seen ophthalmoscopically.
There are often other generalized signs of CNS dysfunction (such as clonus) and cranial deformity.

DIFFERENTIAL DIAGNOSIS

Other conditions of the CNS causing blindness and mydriasis but with intact pupillary light reflexes, for example, cerebral hemorrhage, cerebral vascular accidents, encephalitis, and brain tumors. However, congenital hydrocephalus occurs in very young animals and is associated with characteristic cranial deformities and radiographic changes.

TREATMENT

None is likely to restore vision.

ACQUIRED VISUAL IMPAIRMENT—ACUTE ONSET

Glaucoma

Glaucoma is a pathological increase in intraocular pressure (IOP) that, in animals, is caused by obstructed drainage of aqueous humor from the anterior chamber. Glaucoma may be a primary entity or secondary to other ocular disease. Secondary glaucomas are the most common type encountered in veterinary practice.

Primary Glaucoma

Etiology of the primary glaucomas is poorly understood; the term implies that the pressure increase is a primary event without precedent or concurrent predisposing ocular disease. The condition is classified based upon the gonioscopic appearance of the iridocorneal angle either as open or as narrowed or closed. The current terminology is not totally appropriate because of the anatomy of the carnivore outflow pathways; the ciliary cleft and iridocorneal angle are best evaluated independently.

Glaucomas are classified as to duration as being either *acute* or *chronic*. This is a clinically meaningful categorization because of prognostic significance.

Congenital or Juvenile Glaucoma

This is caused by anomalous mesodermal differentiation of the iridocorneal (filtration) angle (goniodysgenesis) or by more severe anterior segment malformations (anterior segment dysgenesis). Severe cases are born with enlarged, glaucomatous eyes, or *buphthalmos*. We prefer to use the term for eyes enlarged by congenital glaucoma, using *hydrophthalmos* or *megaloglobus* to describe enlargement occurring with glaucoma acquired later in life.

Mild cases of goniodysgenesis have sheets or bands of mesodermal tissue spanning the ciliary cleft and thus reducing aqueous drainage. These cases are often born with apparently normal eyes, but may develop glaucoma in later life. The condition may be seen in any breed but is more common in the Basset Hound, Bouvier des Flandres, and English Cocker Spaniel (recessively inherited).

Primary Open-Angle Glaucoma

Drainage from the anterior chamber is impeded within the trabecular meshwork due to unknown causes. Open-angle glaucoma may be heritable, as seen in the Beagle (recessive trait) and the Siamese cat, or sporadically occurring.

Primary Closed-Angle Glaucoma

This is the most common type of primary glaucoma in the dog. It results from a narrowed iridocorneal angle that eventually closes due to forward movement of the iris, collapse of the ciliary cleft, and formation of peripheral anterior synechiae. It is inherited in the American Cocker Spaniel (recessive), Welsh Springer Spaniel (dominant), Samoyed Miniature Poodle, and Siberian Husky breeds.

Primary glaucoma is usually a bilateral condition, although the second eye may become glaucomatous several months to years after the first eye. Most primary glaucoma cases seen in practice have an hereditary basis.

Secondary Glaucoma

Secondary glaucomas arise as a result of some other ocular disease causing obstruction of aqueous flow either at the pupil or the iridocorneal angle. In veterinary practice this is the most common type of glaucoma, and the most frequent cause of it is lens luxation. Other etiologies include anterior uveitis, ocular trauma, and neoplasia.

CLINICAL SIGNS OF ACUTE GLAUCOMA

Almost all cases of glaucoma in the dog present with acute elevation of IOP, usually greater than 50 mm Hg. This may be a characteristic of the disease in this species, or, more likely, milder elevations are subclinical and go undetected. The primary open-angle glaucomas are more likely to have a slowly progressive clinical course.

The cat is somewhat different; glaucoma may have a more insidious onset. Even with acute disease, the clinical signs may be subtle, consisting of epiphora, mild episcleral injection, and a somewhat dilated pupil with sluggish PLR.

CLINICAL FINDINGS OF ACUTE GLAUCOMA

Pain, blepharospasm, and excessive lacrimation (usually unilateral)

Congestion of episcleral blood vessels (a "red eye")

Corneal edema if the intraocular pressure (IOP) is very high

The pupil is dilated or semidilated with a poor or absent pupillary light reflex (Figure 4–11).

Vision in the acutely affected eye may be present, but is markedly impaired due to the blepharospasm and severe pain experienced by the animal.

Raised IOP. Mechanical tonometry is essential; normal IOP in the dog is 15 to 30 mm Hg.

Papilledema with or without optic disk and peripapillary hemorrhage

In congenital or juvenile glaucoma, gonioscopy of the eye will reveal goniodysgenesis, for example, sheets of pigmented mesodermal tissue spanning the ciliary cleft and impeding aqueous drainage. This is present in both eyes and both eyes should be examined, although gonioscopy in the glaucomatous eye may be impossible if severe corneal edema is present. In primary open-angle

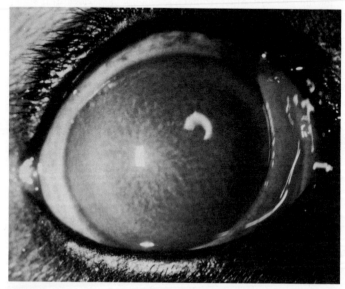

FIGURE 4–11. Acute congestive glaucoma in the right eye of an American Cocker Spaniel.

glaucoma, morphology of the outflow pathways will be unremarkable.

In primary closed-angle glaucoma, gonioscopy will reveal a closed angle in the affected eye and a narrowed angle in the nonglaucomatous eye. Primary open-angle glaucoma does not present initially as an acute congestive glaucoma. It is a more chronic disease with only a slight increase in IOP and gradual loss of vision, with possible acute congestive glaucoma as a late manifestation.

In cases of glaucoma secondary to lens luxation, with focal illumination, the dislocated lens may be visible in the anterior chamber, causing a characteristic focal subcentral corneal opacity with obscuration of the pupil. If the dislocation is posterior, an aphakic crescent will be visualized. The fellow eye may show evidence of lens subluxation, such as iridodonesis (trembling of the iris), a deepened anterior chamber and scalloped iris (due to loss of support by the lens), and vitreal "tags" in the pupil. Terrier breeds are predisposed.

If glaucoma is secondary to anterior uveitis, the iris is usually thickened and spongy in appearance, synechiae may be visible between iris and lens or iris and cornea, and aqueous flare, keratic precipitates, or even hypopyon may also be present.

In cases of glaucoma secondary to ocular trauma, a wide variety of additional signs may be seen, including conjunctival and scleral hemorrhage, lacerations of the globe and adnexa, hyphema, and vitreal hemorrhage.

If glaucoma is secondary to intraocular neoplasia, ciliary body and iris adenomas, adenocarcinomas, and melanomas are the most likely cause. These may be seen as pigmented or nonpigmented masses invading the iridocorneal angle or pushing anteriorly the base of the iris to occlude the filtration angle. Occasionally the tumor may not be visible, but suspicion of this etiology should be aroused by the presence of a focal bulge at the base of the iris and/or equatorial staphylomata. Transillumination may also help to detect a tumor in these cases. Acute glaucoma in the cat is accompanied by less dramatic signs than in the dog; mild episcleral injection and epiphora may be the only presenting signs.

DIFFERENTIATING ACUTE AND CHRONIC GLAUCOMA

Diagnosis of chronic glaucoma is not difficult; one commonly observes:

Enlargement of the globe with equatorial scleral thinning
Variable episcleral injection
Variable corneal edema; occasionally with linear breaks in Descemet's membrane (striate keratopathy)

Secondary lens dislocation (usually posterior) and cataract

Optic atrophy with or without cupping with peripapillary hyperpigmentation and diffuse retinal thinning with tapetal hyperreflectivity and mild retinal vascular attenuation

DIFFERENTIAL DIAGNOSIS OF ACUTE GLAUCOMA

Acute conjunctivitis and acute anterior uveitis are the two main differential diagnoses. With acute conjunctivitis, only the superficial conjunctival blood vessels are congested, not the deeper episcleral vessels. By moving the upper lid manually in various directions, the conjunctival vessels are seen to move with the lid and thus can be differentiated from the immovable episcleral vessels. Similarly, 10% phenylephrine drops applied topically will constrict only the engorged conjunctival vessels. In acute conjunctivitis, the pupillary light reflexes are normal, the IOP is not raised, and there is no corneal edema. Mucopurulent discharge is usually present. With acute anterior uveitis, the pupil tends to be constricted rather than semidilated. The IOP is lowered. The iris appears thickened and spongy, and synechiae may be seen.

PROGNOSIS

The prognosis for vision in acute congestive glaucoma cases in veterinary practice is always guarded; markedly elevated IOP will cause significant irreversible damage to the retina and optic nerve within 48 to 72 hours. In chronic glaucoma, prognosis for vision is poor, and therapy is directed to obtaining and maintaining a cosmetic globe.

Primary glaucoma is a bilateral disease, although rarely concomitantly so. Fellow eyes should be examined critically and followed carefully.

TREATMENT

In the primary glaucomas, medical treatment may be attempted with a combination of an oral carbonic anhydrase inhibitor (dichlorphenamide is effective and well tolerated in dogs at 10 mg/kg BID, and cats at 25 mg BID) to reduce IOP. If the IOP is extremely high, the animal may benefit from administration of an hyperosmotic agent such as 10% mannitol IV (1 gm/kg), oral isosorbide (1 gm/kg), or glycerin (0.5 ml/kg).

With all medical treatments, the IOP should be monitored and gonioscopy performed at regular intervals. If a normal IOP cannot be maintained, or the iridocorneal angle shows progressive narrowing or increasing areas of closure, then surgical intervention is necessary. Indeed, surgery may be said to be indicated in any case of angle-closure glaucoma because medical control at best is temporary. The philosophy of the editor (RLP) is that medical therapy in the great majority of canine and feline patients is useful only in attempting to lower IOP immediately prior to surgery. Glaucoma medication is expensive, has significant side effects, and is just not effective in controlling IOP and preserving vision over a long period of time.

A variety of filtration procedures may be performed in the dog, including corneoscleral trephination with peripheral iridectomy; combined posterior sclerotomy, cyclodialysis, and iridencleisis; laser trabeculoplasty; and gonioimplants. At the present time success rates are not excellent, but certain procedures performed by skilled surgeons may approach acceptable success rates. If the animal is presented with an enlarged hydrophthalmic globe (in which may be seen secondary lens luxation, retinal degeneration, and optic disc cupping), then vision is hopelessly lost. These globes are prone to exposure keratitis and usually associated with some degree of discomfort. Treatment in these cases should be either enucleation (Figure 4–12) or cyclocryotherapy (Figure 4–13), cyclodiathermy, or laser cyclodestruction; evisceration with insertion of an intraocular prosthesis (Figure 4–14); or intravitreal injection of cyclotoxic doses of gentamicin (Figure 4–15). The last three procedures destroy the ciliary body, the site of aqueous production. These procedures are compared and contrasted in Table 4–1.

In cases of glaucoma secondary to lens luxation, surgical removal of the dislocated lens should be performed as soon as possible to prevent permanent damage to the eye and loss of vision. Cases of lens subluxation are also best treated surgically at the time of presentation rather than waiting for the lens to fully luxate and relying on the owner to present the animal. Intracapsular lens extraction accompanied by anterior vitrectomy will in most cases normalize IOP. Retinal detachment and persistence or recurrence of the glaucoma are the most common complications of the surgery.

Glaucoma secondary to anterior uveitis is challenging to treat. Corticosteroids (topical and systemic) to control the uveitis can be used in addition to the usual glaucoma therapeutic agents of a carbonic anhydrase inhibitor (dichlorphenamide) and a topical hypotensive (in dogs there is little evidence that corticosteroids significantly raise IOP). Atropine usage is controversial but indicated if synechiae are extensive. If significant posterior synechiae and iris bombé are present, prompt surgical intervention is necessary to save the eye.

In cases of glaucoma secondary to ocular trauma, resolution of glaucoma may or may not occur, depending on the degree of damage to the globe. Medical treatment may be attempted initially, but surgery may become necessary if the raised IOP cannot be controlled in this way.

Enucleation is advised in glaucomatous eyes with confirmation

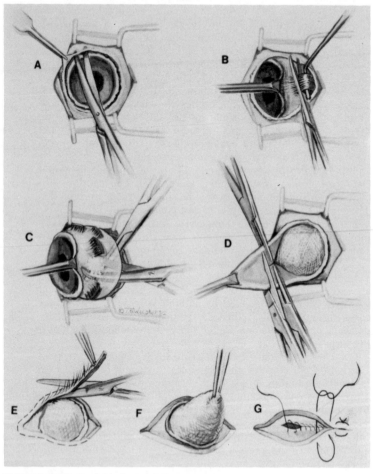

FIGURE 4-12. *See legend on opposite page.*

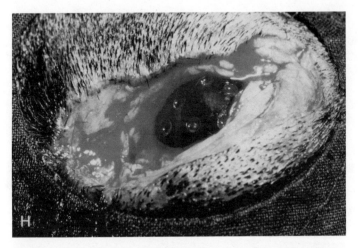

FIGURE 4-12. Subconjunctival enucleation. *A*, A 360° perilimbal conjunctival incision is made and subconjunctival dissection is continued with scissors. *B*, The extraocular muscles are isolated and transected at their insertions on the globe. Intraoperative hemorrhage will be minimal if all sharp dissection is done adjacent to the sclera. *C*, The optic nerve and associated vessels are clamped, ligated, and transected. *D*, After the orbit is packed with gauze, the nictitating membrane is retracted and excised. *E*, Two to 3 mm of eyelid margin are excised. *F*, The gauze packing is removed. *G*, The conjunctiva is closed in a continuous pattern, and then the skin is closed with interrupted mattress sutures.

H, Alternately, a polymethylmethacrylate (PMMA) orbital prosthesis (20 mm in an adult dog or cat) may be inserted to prevent a "shrunken orbit" postoperatively. Adequate closure of deep tissues over the implant is important for success. Orbital hydromucoceles with drainage is the most commonly encountered complication. These should be explored surgically, the walls excised, and the prosthesis (if used) removed. From Peiffer RL Jr, et al: Surgery of the canine & feline orbit, adnexa, and globe. Part I: Introduction, instrumentation, and surgery of the orbit. *Companion Animal Practice* 1:20–34, July 1987.

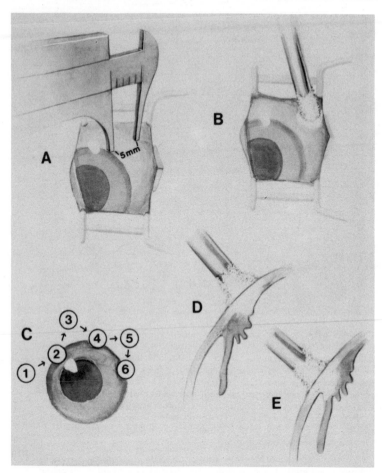

FIGURE 4-13. Cyclocryosurgery. Liquid nitrogen, nitrous oxide, or carbon dioxide may be utilized. *A*, A caliper is used to identify a point 5 mm posterior to the limbus directly over the pars plicata of the ciliary body. *B*, The cryoprobe is applied for two one-minute freezes at each site. *C–E*, The probe positions form an olympic ring pattern, alternating sites over the ciliary body *D*, and the iridocorneal angle *E*, for a minimum of 180°. Complications include postoperative edema and uveitis; exudative retinal detachment; continued elevation of IOP; and corneoscleral necrosis and/or phthisis bulbus due to overfreezing. The technique tends to be difficult to control and is somewhat unpredictable. From Peiffer RL Jr, et al: Surgery of the canine and feline orbit, adnexa, and glove. Part VIII. *Companion Animal Practice* 2:3–15, February 1988.

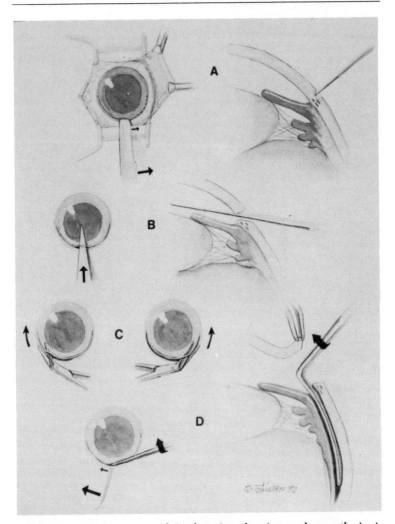

FIGURE 4-14. Eviscemation with implantation of an intraocular prosthesis. *A*, Following a lateral canthotomy, a half-thickness 180° corneoscleral incision is made with a #64 Beaver blade. *B*, The anterior chamber is entered with a #65 Beaver blade. *C*, The incision is completed with curved corneoscleral scissors. *D*, A cyclodialysis spatula is inserted directly under the sclera and rotated to detach the iris and ciliary body. From Peiffer RL Jr, et al: Surgery of the canine and feline orbit, adnexa, and glove. Part VIII. *Companion Animal Practice* 2:3–15, February 1988.

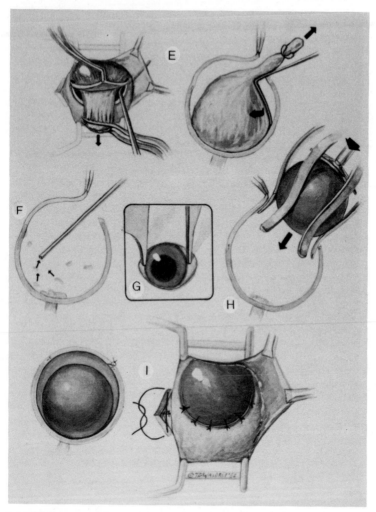

FIGURE 4-14. Implantation of an intraocular prosthesis (continued). *E*, The iris is grasped with capsule forceps and traction is applied while using the spatula to complete removal of the uveal tissue and the enclosed intraocular contents. These tissues should be submitted for histopathologic study. Care must be taken to avoid damage to the endothelial surface of the cornea, which would result in possible ulceration or a less cosmetic result. *F*, Significant hemorrhage is to be expected, and suction is useful for hemostasis and to identify and remove remaining vestiges of tissue. *G*, The fellow eye is measured with a caliper prior to surgery, and a silastic sphere selected which is one mm larger than the horizontal corneal diameter. *H*, A sphere introducer is used for placement of the

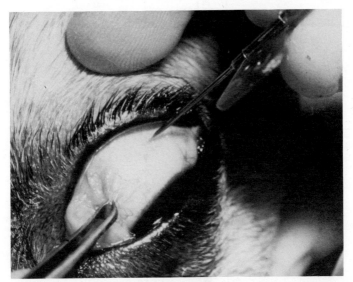

FIGURE 4-15. Intravitreal injection of gentamicin. Usually the procedure can be performed with only topical anesthesia; sedation or short-acting anesthesia may be used in uncooperative patients. The fornices are cleansed with half-strength povidone iodine solution, the lids held open by speculum or an assistant, and the globe stabilized by grasping superior conjunctiva with small-toothed forceps. At the 12 o'clock position, a 20-gauge butterfly infusion needle is inserted 6–8 mm posterior to the limbus, directed toward the posterior pole to a depth of 10 mm, while continuing to stabilize both globe and butterfly. Then 0.5 ml of vitreous, which in these globes will be liquefied and readily aspirated, is removed; 0.25 ml of 100 mg/ml gentamicin (25 mg) and 0.25 ml of a 4 mg/ml dexamethasone (1 mg) solution are injected and the needle removed. Topical antibiotics and corticosteroids are prescribed postoperatively.

Complications include trauma to the lens capsule with lens-induced uveitis if the needle is misdirected, intraocular hemorrhage, cataract, persistent elevated IOP (the injection may be repeated), or phthisis bulbus. The procedure is contraindicated in chronically glaucomatous eyes with suspicion of an intraocular tumor. It is a safe, inexpensive method to manage blind, glaucomatous eyes.

---

sphere within the eviscerated globe. *I*, Routine closure is completed using 7-0 Vicryl to suture the corneoscleral incision and a two-layered closure of the canthotomy incision. Complications include predictable transient postoperative inflammation, which is controlled with topical corticosteroids, and occasional rejection of the prosthesis associated with wound dehiscence or corneal ulceration. Prosthesis extrusion may occur in the presence of regrowth of an intraocular tumor; suspicion of a tumor or active infection are contraindications for the procedure.

TABLE 4-1. Comparison of Alternatives in the Treatment of Chronic Glaucoma

	GENERAL ANESTHESIA	EXPENSE	PREDICTABILITY	POSTOPERATIVE AFTERCARE	COSMESIS
Pharmacologic Ablation	+/−	Inexpensive	++	+	+/−
Cyclocryosurgery	+	Moderate	+	++	+/−
Intraocular Prosthesis	+	Costly	++	++	+
Enucleation	+	Moderate	+++	−	−

or strong suspicion of intraocular tumor to both relieve pain and avert the risk of tumor metastases or local invasion.

Cornea

CAV I or CAV II Uveitis/Corneal Edema

Keratouveitis in the dog may be caused by infectious canine hepatitis (ICH) either due to natural infection with canine adenovirus type I (CAV I) or postvaccination reactions to live CAV I or rarely CAV II. It has become uncommon in dogs with the advent of CAV II vaccines and the greater use of inactivated adenovirus vaccines.

CLINICAL FINDINGS

Vision is only slightly affected in the acute phase due to bilateral mild uveitis with conjunctivitis and photophobia.

Some dogs, however, go on to develop severe uveitis 7 to 21 days after infection or vaccination: IOP is low and vision is grossly impaired due to keratic precipitates and hypopyon, which may occlude the pupil, and accompanying corneal edema ("blue eye").

Corneal edema is usually unilateral and progresses from the limbus towards the central cornea.

If corneal edema is particularly intense, the eye may also show *keratoconus* (a conical bulging of the central cornea), *bullous keratopathy* (small fluid-filled blisters of the corneal epithelium), and keratitis with corneal neovascularization.

Glaucoma is an occasional sequel to the severe uveitis (usually unilateral).

DIFFERENTIAL DIAGNOSIS

Acute glaucoma: IOP is raised in glaucoma, not lowered. It is rarely accompanied by uveitis with hypopyon and keratic precipitates. There is no history of ICH or recent vaccination with CAV I/CAV II.

Corneal endothelial dystrophy: IOP is usually normal, and the eyes are fairly comfortable. There is no evidence of keratouveitis and no history of ICH or recent vaccination. Endothelial dystrophies often show a breed incidence (Chihuahua, Boston Terrier) with a chronic progressive onset in older animals.

Corneal edema accompanying anterior lens luxation: IOP tends to be raised, and the corneal edema is usually initially focal and subcentral. There is a breed incidence (terriers) and no history of ICH or recent vaccination.

Corneal Ulceration or Perforation

Corneal ulceration and perforation are immediate causes of visual impairment because of the pain, blepharospasm, protrusion of the third eyelid, corneal edema, surface irregularity, ocular discharge, and, with perforation, anterior synechiae and sometimes collapse of the globe. However, pain is the predominant sign, and these conditions are discussed in detail in a later chapter.

CLINICAL FINDINGS

Pain, blepharospasm, excessive lacrimation, sometimes purulent ocular discharge

Defects in integrity of corneal epithelium and stroma (use focal oblique light source and confirm by using fluorescein)

Accompanying corneal edema, cellular infiltration, and vascularization

There may be an associated anterior uveitis with or without hypopyon.

If perforated, pigmented iris tissue is usually visible within the corneal lesion forming anterior synechiae. Protruded tissue is usually covered by a gray fibrinous membrane.

DIFFERENTIAL DIAGNOSIS

Corneal opacity associated with congenital anterior synechiae: the eye is comfortable and the corneal epithelium is intact. A persistent pupillary membrane is visible attaching to the iris collarette.

Corneal scar: dense white corneal opacity in a comfortable eye. The corneal epithelium is intact.

Corneal abscess, corneal tumor: uncommon, raised masses on the corneal surface

Chemical Burns

Acid and alkali burns of the cornea are both serious. Alkali burns in particular can cause rapid corneal opacification with visual impairment and even perforation of the globe. Sight-threatening complications include corneal perforation, symblepharon formation, uveitis, and secondary glaucoma.

CLINICAL FINDINGS

Pain, blepharospasm, excessive lacrimation

Corneal epithelium is destroyed.

Depending on the case, the corneal stroma is also variably destroyed and appears melted, edematous, and opaque.

Conjunctiva often appears white.

TREATMENT AND PROGNOSIS

Prompt and copious irrigation and supportive treatment as required. Prognosis for vision is usually guarded.

Anterior Segment

Anterior Uveitis

Anterior uveitis is an important cause of acute visual impairment, particularly bilateral severe cases; it is discussed in detail in the chapter on abnormal appearance.

CLINICAL FINDINGS

Pain, blepharospasm, photophobia, excessive lacrimation
Pupil is constricted.
Iris is thickened, iris vasculature engorged, and, with chronicity, the iris is discolored.
Aqueous flare and keratic precipitates are often visible.
Hypopyon can be present and may even fill the anterior chamber in exceptionally severe cases.
Perilimbal corneal vascularization and sometimes corneal edema
Episcleral congestion
Lowered intraocular pressure

Hyphema

Hyphema, that is, blood in the anterior chamber, may occasionally cause acute visual loss. Hyphema may follow trauma to the anterior uvea, but it may also reflect sight-threatening diseases of the posterior segment, including retinal detachments and hemorrhage associated with blood-clotting disorders or systemic hypertension. Permanent loss of vision may result from sequelae including uveitis, glaucoma, synechiae, and cataracts.

Lipid-Laden Aqueous Humor

This is a rare cause of visual impairment. The appearance of the eye may be altered dramatically. Affected animals may show little evidence of visual embarrassment due to the presence of lipids in the ocular media, but anterior uveitis is often present and may accordingly cause some loss of vision.

Cataracts

Cataracts generally cause visual impairment after chronic progression (usually over months to years). Cataracts that can cause acute visual loss due to rapid progression tend to be those associated with diabetes mellitus or trauma. Cataracts due to certain toxic agents develop rapidly, but these are rarely encountered in practice.

Vitreous

Vitreous Hemorrhage

ETIOLOGY

Vitreous hemorrhage may be associated with trauma, systemic hypertension, clotting deficiencies, or neoplasia. Occasional cases are spontaneous and idiopathic.

Trauma

The most common causes of vitreous hemorrhage are blunt trauma to the head or globe and penetrating injuries to the eye. The hemorrhage originates usually from retinal blood vessels but may also involve the uveal vasculature.

CLINICAL FINDINGS

Usually, but not always, unilateral

Blood is present within the vitreous body and obscures much of the fundus.

There may be accompanying hyphema.

In the case of penetrating foreign bodies (most commonly gun pellets), the tract may be outlined by red blood cells; an entry wound can sometimes be detected as a corneal lesion or bulbar conjunctival hemorrhage and bruising.

A foreign body may be visible in the vitreous or it may have passed through the globe; an exit wound is sometimes visible ophthalmoscopically.

DIAGNOSIS

On the basis of the clinical findings and history of trauma

X-rays may help to detect a foreign body in the orbit.

TREATMENT

There is no treatment for traumatic vitreous hemorrhage. If accompanied by anterior uveitis, it should be treated with topical atropine and corticosteroids.

PROGNOSIS AND SEQUELAE

The blood will clot and may take many months to resorb without untoward effects; "floaters" may remain. Possible sequelae include glaucoma, traction retinal detachment, and vitreous syneresis.

Systemic Hypertension

Usually associated with chronic renal disease, adrenal tumors, or hypothyroidism, this may cause exudative retinal detachment, retinal hemorrhages, and intravitreal hemorrhage in the dog and cat.

CLINICAL FINDINGS

Usually bilateral. Therefore, the fellow eye should be examined for signs of retinopathy.
Sudden onset of blindness
Exudative retinal detachment, intraretinal and preretinal hemorrhages
Often, but not always, systemic signs associated with the underlying disease process

DIAGNOSIS

On the basis of the clinical findings
Blood biochemistry for organ function
Measurement of blood pressure

TREATMENT

Treat the hypertension with diuretics, dietary control, and/or vasodilators and the primary condition if possible. The prognosis for return of vision improves with early treatment.

Coagulopathies

Coagulopathies are an important differential diagnosis in cases of vitreous hemorrhage and include thrombocytopenia, hyperviscosity syndrome and other blood dyscrasias and warfarin poisoning.

CLINICAL FINDINGS

Often bilateral ocular hemorrhage including retinal and preretinal hemorrhages
If the retinal vasculature can be visualized, it may appear anemic.
Hemorrhages on the mucous membranes, skin, and elsewhere on the body
Pale mucous membranes

DIAGNOSIS

Clinical signs
Hematology

TREATMENT

Treat the primary condition.

Intraocular Tumor

Both primary and secondary intraocular tumors may present with vitreous hemorrhage.

CLINICAL FINDINGS

Unilateral vitreous hemorrhage in the case of primary intraocular tumors

May be bilateral vitreous hemorrhages in lymphosarcoma (often with retinal detachment and hemorrhages) or metastatic carcinomas

Ciliary body epithelial tumors and anterior uveal melanomas usually involve the anterior uveal tract and tend to distort the pupil and/or cause a focal bulging forward of the iris.

Mydriatic drops may be required in order to visualize a mass in the posterior segment.

Use transillumination to confirm that the tissue swelling is a solid mass rather than a detachment or cystic structure.

Lymphosarcoma frequently involves the anterior segment and aqueous humor.

If the ocular neoplasm is a secondary tumor, there may be systemic signs of neoplasia, such as enlarged lymph nodes.

DIAGNOSIS

On the findings of careful ocular examination including transillumination

Hematology and systemic signs in secondary neoplastic cases

Vitreous or aqueous paracentesis to obtain specimens for cytological examination

TREATMENT

Enucleation if primary intraocular tumor
Euthanasia or chemotherapy if lymphosarcoma

Vitreous Inflammation

The vitreous is an avascular structure that cannot mount an active inflammatory response. However, the vitreous is often involved passively in inflammations of surrounding tissues (chorioretinitis and optic neuritis), wherein inflammatory cells migrate into the vitreous body. The most severe and serious inflammatory process involving the vitreous is the vitreous abscess or endophthalmitis, which usually follows foreign body perforation of the globe.

CLINICAL FINDINGS

Vitreous haze, due to inflammatory cells, causes blurring of fundus detail.

Areas of active chorioretinitis or optic neuritis may be seen.

In the case of foreign bodies and vitreous abscessation, a yellow mass is seen behind the lens and the eye is congested, inflamed, and painful.

DIAGNOSIS

On the basis of the clinical findings

If vitreous abscessation is present, then vitreous paracentesis should be performed and the aspirate examined and cultured to determine antibiotic sensitivities of any micro-organisms involved.

DIFFERENTIAL DIAGNOSIS

Other causes of vitreous opacification and leukocoria include:

Cataract: lens is opaque; eye is not usually inflamed.

Total retinal detachment: retinal blood vessels are clearly visible, often on the posterior surface of the lens; the eye is blind and not inflamed.

PHPV: congenital condition; a plaque of fibrovascular tissue is present on the posterior lens capsule and the eye is not inflamed.

Asteroid hyalosis: spherical white bodies are suspended in gelled vitreous, and the eye is not inflamed.

Synchisis scintillans: glittering angular crystals are freely mobile in liquified vitreous, and the eye is not inflamed.

PROGNOSIS

In mild cases, associated with chorioretinitis and/or optic neuritis, prognosis depends on the severity of the underlying tissue inflammation; widespread chorioretinitis or optic neuritis may result in optic atrophy and blindness. Effective therapy may limit the disease process. However, vitreous syneresis (liquefaction) is a possible sequel that may predispose the eye to retinal detachment.

In severe cases with vitreous abscessation, prognosis is poor. Effective therapy rarely saves vision but may prevent phthisis bulbi.

TREATMENT

In mild cases, use antibiotic and corticosteroid therapy (topical and systemic).

In severe cases, depending on the results of vitreous paracentesis, inject subconjunctival gentamicin (0.5 ml) and treat with systemic, broad-spectrum antibiotics. Oculomycoses may be the cause, and treatment may be attempted with systemic antifungals.

Retina

Sudden Acquired Retinal Degeneration (SARD)

This is a recently described condition in the dog in which affected animals develop sudden blindness due to rapid photoreceptor degeneration. The etiology is unknown, although a toxic cause has been suggested.

CLINICAL FINDINGS

Sudden blindness (over days)

Bilaterally dilated, unresponsive pupils

Affected dogs are usually middle-aged and in fairly good health.

May be evidence of subclinical hepatic or Cushing's disease

Ophthalmoscopy initially reveals a normal fundus in both eyes; however, reexamination several weeks later reveals classical signs of generalized retinal degeneration (hyperreflectivity, vessel attenuation) and, later, optic atrophy.

The retinal degeneration is progressive.

DIAGNOSIS

On the basis of the history and clinical findings

Electroretinography reveals an extinguished ERG.

DIFFERENTIAL DIAGNOSIS

Classical optic neuritis: ophthalmoscopy reveals a swollen, edematous optic disk and engorged retinal blood vessels, sometimes with papillary and peripapillary hemorrhages, retinal edema, and/or detachment.

Retrobulbar optic neuritis: ophthalmoscopy reveals a normal fundus as in early SARD cases, but the ERG is normal or only mildly abnormal in optic neuritis.

Central blindness (due to cerebral trauma or stroke): there are usually other signs of CNS involvement. Ophthalmoscopy several weeks later does not show retinal atrophy. The ERG is normal.

PROGNOSIS

Hopeless. Blindness is total and irreversible.

TREATMENT

None.

Retinal Detachment

Retinal detachments are not infrequently a cause of sudden visual loss. They may be classified into three types: exudative (serous), tractional, and rhegmatogenous (perforated). In retinal detachments the neurosensory retina, including the photoreceptors, separates from the retinal pigment epithelium along the boundary between the two layers of the primitive optic cup. Separation of the rods and cones from their vascular supply—the choriocapillaris—will result in irreversible photoreceptor degeneration over a period of several weeks.

Exudative Detachments

The most common form of retinal detachment seen in veterinary practice, exudative detachments result from fluid of uveal vasculature origin accumulating between the photoreceptors and the retinal pigment epithelium. The retina becomes elevated as flat or bullous detachments and may progress to total retinal detachment, sometimes with disinsertion or dialysis (tearing of the retinal attachments at the ora ciliaris retinae) (Figure 4–16).

ETIOLOGY

Hypertension: chronic renal disease, adrenal tumors, or hypothyroidism may result in hypertension, causing bilateral serous retinal detachments with or without associated intraocular hemorrhage.

Infection: choroiditis or chorioretinitis (canine distemper, feline infectious peritonitis, feline leukemia-lymphosarcoma, oculomycoses, toxoplasmosis) may result in exudative retinal detachment.

Immune-mediated inflammation: seen in Akitas and other breeds with immune-mediated uveitis

Trauma: insult to the globe may elicit a focal scleritis with localized choroiditis and edema, resulting in focal exudative retinal detachment.

CLINICAL FINDINGS

Often sudden-onset loss of vision, especially if bilateral

If unilateral, the condition may not be detected except on ophthalmoscopy.

Partial retinal detachments (flat or bullous) appear ophthalmoscopically as elevated areas that are out of focus compared to the optic disk and focus at positive diopter settings on the instrument.

If the detachment is complete, the retina may be seen, with focal illumination, as a veil-like structure lying against the posterior surface of the lens or moving in the vitreous.

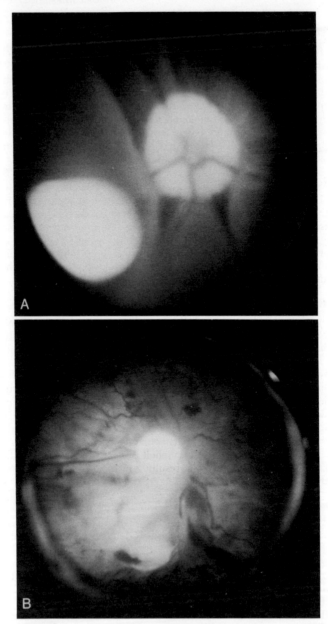

FIGURE 4–16. *See legend on opposite page.*

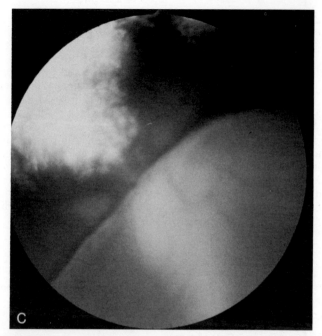

FIGURE 4-16. Retinal detachment. *A*, Exudative detachment in a German Shepherd with immune-mediated posterior uveitis. The retina is seen as a fold of tissue billowing forward from its attachment at the optic disk. *B*, Exudative detachment in a cat with feline infectious peritonitis; numerous retinal hemorrhages are also seen within the retrolental, totally detached retina. *C*, Idiopathic rhegmatogenous detachment in a Boston Terrier. The superior retina is torn at the ora and draped over the optic disk.

Retinal blood vessels over a retinal detachment are tortuous.

Retinal and intravitreal hemorrhages may be present due to vasculitis, tearing of the detached retina, or neovascularization.

If the retina is totally detached, the pupil is dilated, but a pupillary light reflex may still be present for several days to weeks after detachment.

DIAGNOSIS

Ophthalmoscopic appearance

May be accompanying signs of systemic illness (hematology, blood biochemistry)

DIFFERENTIAL DIAGNOSIS

Retinal detachments due to other causes (postoperative or congenital; CEA, retinal dysplasia): the immediate history of the case and age of the animal aid in differentiation.

Other causes of leukocoria ("white pupil"): cataracts, PHPV, endophthalmitis, organized intraocular hemorrhage, posterior segment neoplasia

PROGNOSIS

Exudative retinal detachments (even if total) can reattach and the photoreceptors regenerate if the retina has not been detached for too long; if the retina remains detached for several weeks, then visual loss is usually permanent. Prognosis will also depend on any underlying disease process, for example, if hypertension or renal disease can be treated and controlled. Detachments due to focal choroidal inflammation or trauma have a good prognosis for reattachment.

TREATMENT

Conservative. Treat exudative retinal detachments with diuretics to enhance removal of subretinal fluid and with systemic corticosteroids to control inflammation and immune-mediated responses. Treat any underlying disease if possible.

Traction Retinal Detachments

Vitreoretinal adhesions, preretinal membranes, and/or traction bands contract and mechanically detach the retina.

ETIOLOGY

Postintraocular surgery
After perforating ocular injuries and/or vitreous hemorrhage

CLINICAL FINDINGS

Usually unilateral
Retina is detached with tortuous retinal blood vessels (as described under exudative retinal detachments).
White traction bands may be seen ophthalmoscopically.

DIAGNOSIS

History and ophthalmoscopic appearance
No evidence of systemic illness

PROGNOSIS

Traction retinal detachments are serious and tend to be permanent.

TREATMENT

Medical treatment is of no use. Intraocular microsurgery can be used to section traction bands, but the equipment required for such surgery is not available to most veterinarians.

Rhegmatogenous Retinal Detachments

These detachments are caused by full-thickness retinal holes or tears and are uncommon in veterinary practice, in contrast with the situation in humans. The vitreous must also be liquefied (undergone syneresis) in order for the retina to detach. The liquefied vitreous percolates through the retinal hole and gradually elevates the retina and extends the subretinal space.

ETIOLOGY

Some cases of CEA and retinal dysplasia

Atrophic, following chorioretinal inflammatory or degenerative atrophy

Spontaneous; giant peripheral tears have been seen to occur without precedent ocular disease.

Traumatic, following cataract surgery, removal of luxated lenses, or accidental blunt trauma

Some senile canine eyes do have retinal holes, but the retina remains attached as long as the vitreous is not diseased.

CLINICAL FINDINGS

Usually unilateral (sometimes bilateral in CEA or RD cases)

Retina partially or totally detached with or without disinsertion

The vitreous is liquefied so that opacities float about freely in the vitreous with eye movements.

The hole or tear in the retina may be visible ophthalmoscopically, but is often difficult to find. Retinal holes and tears may occur in an already detached retina of the exudative or traction forms.

DIAGNOSIS

The animal's age and breed in the case of CEA or RD

Ophthalmoscopy to detect the presence of a retinal hole or tear and abnormal vitreous

No signs of systemic illness or other ocular disease

PROGNOSIS AND TREATMENT

Prognosis is guarded. These cases are best managed by a specialist. Laser treatment to limit a partial detachment is a remote possibility. Drainage of subretinal fluid, application of a scleral buckle, filling the posterior segment with air, gas, or silicone oil, and creating a cryosurgical scar at the hole or tear can be effective in relatively acute cases with localized holes or tears. Prognosis with giant peripheral tears (greater than 90°) is poor.

Optic Disk

Optic Neuritis

Optic neuritis is an inflammation of the optic nerve, either close to the globe (papillitis, postlaminar optic neuritis) or closer to the brain (retrobulbar or prelaminar optic neuritis). It may be a primary ocular disease or secondary to systemic disease.

ETIOLOGY

Idiopathic (immune-mediated): common
Infectious: canine distemper, oculomycoses
Extension of inflammation from adjacent tissues: ocular, orbital, sinuses, meninges
Neoplastic: reticulosis of the central nervous system, optic nerve tumors
Trauma
Vitamin A deficiency
Toxic: lead, DDT, arsanilic acid poisoning
Pancreatitis

CLINICAL FINDINGS

Bilateral cases usually present with acute-onset blindness (unilateral optic neuritis may go unnoticed).
Widely dilated pupils with absent pupillary light reflexes
Classical papillitis or postlaminar optic neuritis appears ophthalmoscopically as an enlarged, swollen, pink, edematous optic disk with blurred borders and congested, engorged blood vessels that dip down over the elevated rim of the disk; there may or may not be papillary and peripapillary hemorrhages and peripapillary retinal edema, detachment, or folds. Often there is prepapillary vitreous haze due to cellular infiltrates, and other ocular tissues may also be involved (uveitis) (Figure 4–17).
In retrobulbar or prelaminar optic neuritis, ophthalmoscopy reveals a normal optic disk.

DIAGNOSIS

History, clinical findings, and ophthalmoscopic appearance
Electroretinography reveals a normal or minimally affected ERG.

DIFFERENTIAL DIAGNOSIS

Sudden acquired retinal degeneration (SARD) in the dog: the fundus appears normal initially (as in retrobulbar optic neuritis). In SARD the ERG is extinguished.

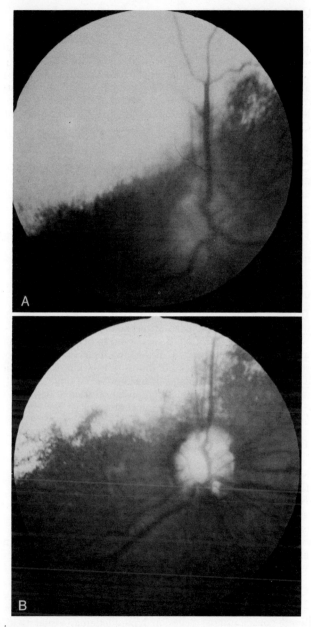

FIGURE 4–17. Idiopathic optic neuritis in a Dachshund. *A,* The optic disk margins are indistinct. *B,* In spite of aggressive corticosteroid therapy, the disease resulted in significant optic atrophy.

Papilledema: the ocular lesion is rarely the reason for presentation of the case. Orbital disease or other signs of CNS disease (due to a space-occupying lesion and/or raised intracranial pressure) are often present. Vision is often normal, unlike optic neuritis.

Central blindness: the fundus is normal and, depending on the level of the CNS lesion, pupillary light reflexes are often intact. Other signs of CNS disease are usually present.

PROGNOSIS

Guarded. Even if treatment is apparently successful and some vision is restored, this can subsequently be lost due to optic atrophy. Rapid response to treatment improves the prognosis.

TREATMENT

High doses of systemic corticosteroids. Prednisolone (4 mg/kg daily) is recommended; continue for several weeks.

Treat any underlying disease (oculomycosis, meningitis).

Central Nervous System

Diseases of the central nervous system can cause acute loss of vision that may be difficult to differentiate from optic neuritis except that other signs of CNS disease tend to be present. Localized brain damage above the level of the lateral geniculate ganglion or rostral colliculus may cause blindness, but pupillary light reflexes are intact. However, damage to the midbrain, either directly or due to compression by expanding cerebral lesions or brain edema, affects the pupillary light reflexes as well as the extraocular muscles.

ETIOLOGY

Trauma

Postanesthetic hypoxia

Inflammation

Toxic hepatic encephalopathy

Cerebral vascular accident

Postictal

Even long-standing, space-occupying brain lesions can herniate and give rise to acute-onset clinical signs including blindness or visual field defects.

CLINICAL FINDINGS: TRAUMA, SOME SPACE-OCCUPYING LESIONS, INFLAMMATION

Altered consciousness, occasional papilledema, visual field defects, or blindness

If tentorial herniation has occurred, there will be signs of vestibular and cerebellar dysfunction, pupils may show miosis followed by mydriasis as intracranial pressure increases, and divergent strabismus and nystagmus are sometimes seen.

A range of other nervous signs may be noticed, including sensory deficits in touch, pain, and proprioception, and motor deficits such as circling, hemiplegia, and hemiparesis.

A common visual field deficit is hemianopia; due to a lesion of the optic tract, optic radiation, or occipital cortex, the animal tends to bump into objects on one side only.

CLINICAL FINDINGS: POSTICTAL

Dogs who have suffered an epileptic fit (perhaps unobserved by the owner) often present with hemianopia or blindness, confusion or impaired consciousness, ataxia, and incontinence.

DIAGNOSIS

Clinical findings of blindness or visual field deficits, intact pupillary light reflexes, a normal fundus or papilledema, optic neuritis, or retinitis, associated with other nervous signs

DIFFERENTIAL DIAGNOSIS

Optic neuritis or SARD: there are no associated signs of CNS disease and the pupils are always fixed and dilated.

PROGNOSIS

Generally guarded. If treatment is instituted promptly and the condition is reversible, then the prognosis for return of vision is improved. Postictal visual loss may also be transient. However, in cases of postanesthesia hypoxia, the brain damage is often irreversible.

TREATMENT

Oxygen and ventilation if necessary. Reduce brain edema with osmotic diuretics (20% mannitol slowly by intravenous injection at 1 to 3 g/kg) and repeated large doses of corticosteroids.

With head injuries, bone fragments should be removed and skull fractures elevated. Systemic antibiosis if the fracture is compound. If deterioration is rapid, then brain decompression by tapping the lateral ventricles is indicated.

ACQUIRED VISUAL LOSS— CHRONIC PROGRESSIVE

Conditions Involving the Globe

Phthisis Bulbi

Phthisis bulbi is a sequel to a severe ocular insult, intraocular inflammation, or degenerative processes within the eye that affect the ciliary body. The resultant reduction or cessation of aqueous production causes a lowering of intraocular pressure and an end-stage shrunken globe with degenerate contents.

CLINICAL FINDINGS

Usually unilateral

Following the insult or inflammation of the ciliary body, the IOP begins to fall and the eye is noticeably soft (compare with fellow eye).

The lowered IOP is followed (over several weeks to months) by gradual shrinkage of the globe and progressive visual impairment (if the original insult to the globe has not already caused blindness).

The end-stage eye is small, shrunken, and totally blind with variable degrees of corneal opacification and vascularization.

PROGNOSIS AND TREATMENT

Phthisical globes are predisposed to recurrent chronic conjunctivitis because of the pooling of ocular secretions; regular irrigation with sterile saline and topical antibiotics as required often maintains reasonable cosmesis. If not, enucleation is recommended. In cats, these globes are predisposed to the development of primary ocular sarcomas, and enucleation is indicated.

Cornea

Corneal Vascularization, Scarring, and Pigmentation

Keratoconjunctivitis Sicca (KCS)

This deficiency of tears may cause acute visual loss due to corneal ulceration and perforation, but more commonly, in advanced cases, it causes a chronic, progressive deterioration in vision due to corneal vascularization, scarring, and pigmentation.

CLINICAL FINDINGS

Unilateral or bilateral

Thick, tenacious, mucopurulent exudates often adhere to the lids or accumulate in the fornices.

The cornea is lusterless, and the conjunctivae are hyperemic and thickened.

As the KCS becomes long-standing, the dry cornea becomes superficially vascularized.

This is followed by patchy corneal pigmentation and scarring.

In advanced cases, the cornea may be densely and completely pigmented with consequent severe visual impairment and even blindness.

Pigmentary Keratitis

This condition is a response of the cornea to chronic irritation and/or inflammation in which superficial vascularization is followed by deposition of melanin in the corneal epithelium and anterior stroma.

ETIOLOGY

Chronic keratoconjunctivitis sicca
Chronic superficial keratitis (pannus)
Mechanical irritation due to foreign bodies in the conjunctival sac, distichiasis, ectopic cilia, entropion, eyelid scarring, eyelid neoplasia, or trichiasis (most commonly associated with nasal fold irritation)
Exposure keratitis due to lagophthalmos (inability to close the eyelids completely over the cornea), buphthalmos/hydrophthalmos, and exophthalmos

CLINICAL FINDINGS

Bilateral or unilateral, depending on the etiology
Signs associated with the primary condition are found in addition to the corneal vascularization and pigmentation, such as blepharospasm and excessive lacrimation with ectopic cilia and mucopurulent discharge with KCS.
Loss of vision is present, depending on the degree of corneal pigmentation.

DIAGNOSIS AND DIFFERENTIAL DIAGNOSIS

Diagnosing the primary disease is essential.

Keratoconjunctivitis sicca: tenacious mucopurulent discharge is present, sometimes adherent to the lids. The cornea is dry and lusterless, and the conjunctivae thickened and hyperemic. Schirmer tear tests reveal deficient tear production. There may be a breed incidence (Lhasa Apso or West Highland White Terrier) or a history of chronic drug administration (sulfasalazine) for colitis.
Pannus: bilateral, breed (German Shepherd), distribution (temporal quadrants), and appearance (granulation tissue) of lesions are characteristic.
Foreign body: pigmentation tends to be focal. Signs of irritation (blepharospasm, epiphora) are usually present. Search for a foreign body in the conjunctival fornices and behind the third eyelid.
Lid-associated keratitis—distichia, ectopic cilia, entropion, lid scarring, lid neoplasms, and nasal fold irritation (brachycephalic breeds).
Lagophthalmos, that is, inability of the eyelids to protect the

cornea effectively and distribute the tearfilm, results in exposure keratitis and may be related to anatomic or pathologic exophthalmos, buphthalmos, or neurologic disorders. The former is a breed problem (Pekingese, Pug); the globe is normal in size, but the bony orbits are shallow. Buphthalmos or hydrophthalmos is seen in chronic glaucoma with globe enlargement. With neurogenic lagophthalmos, the globe is normal in size, but the orbicularis oculi muscle is paralyzed due to a lesion of the facial nerve (VII). Corneal menace reflexes are absent on the affected side. The cornea may be desensitized due to a lesion of the trigeminal nerve (V). The corneal reflex is absent on the affected side, but the menace reflexes are intact.

TREATMENT

Treat the primary condition first, if possible (restore tear film in KCS; surgically correct nasal folds to alleviate trichiasis [Figure 4-18]; lateral or medial canthoplasty in anatomic exophthalmos and lagophthalmos [Figure 4-19]). Once the primary condition is corrected, topical corticosteroids can be used (in the absence of corneal ulceration) to reduce corneal vascularization. This will also have the effect of reducing corneal pigmentation to a certain degree, thereby improving vision. However, if pigmentation is too dense or corticosteroids prove ineffective, then superficial keratectomy is indicated. The prognosis for restoration of useful vision after superficial keratectomy is good, providing predisposing anatomical and/or physiologic factors are managed.

Pannus

Chronic superficial keratitis or corneal pannus is a condition in which the subepithelial tissues are infiltrated by plasma cells and lymphocytes, granulation tissue (vascularization), and pigmentation. It is a disease primarily of the German Shepherd Dog, but other breeds are also affected, particularly the Greyhound and Border Collie.

ETIOLOGY

There is a breed predisposition in the German Shepherd, most likely involving autoimmune and various irritating factors, including sunlight and/or ultraviolet radiation, dust, and pollen grains.

CLINICAL FINDINGS

It is a bilateral, generally symmetrical disease, usually noticed in dogs three to five years of age.

The earliest changes occur in the *pigment patch,* a normal, heavily pigmented patch of perilimbal bulbar conjunctiva in the inferotemporal quadrant.

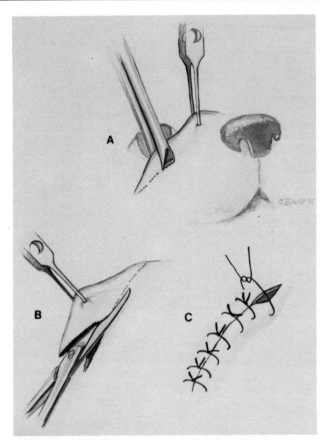

FIGURE 4-18. Excision of nasal folds for medial pigmentary keratitis in brachycephalic breeds. Following routine preparation of the area, the nasal fold is grasped and crimped serially at its base with Allis tissue forceps to delineate the incision (A). The nasal fold is excised with Mayo scissors (B) and the skin apposed with simple interrupted sutures of 4-0 silk with good skin-to-skin apposition (C). Subcutaneous sutures are not necessary. From Peiffer RL Jr et al: Surgery of the canine and feline orbit, adnexa, and globe. Part II: Congenital abnormalities of the eyelid and cilia abnormalities. *Companion Animal Practice* 1:27–38, August 1987.

Depigmentation and follicle formation are evident in the pigment patch, with focal edema and granulation tissue.

Superficial vascularization of the cornea begins in the inferotemporal quadrant of each eye and progressively extends across

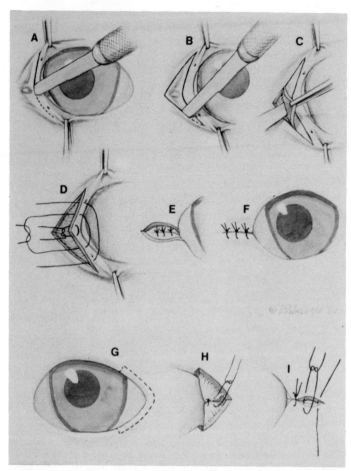

FIGURE 4–19. Permanent medial (*A–F*) and lateral (*G–I*) canthoplasty. Lateral canthoplasty is indicated for pigmentary keratitis associated with anatomic exophthalmos and lagophthalmos; medial canthoplasty for hairy caruncle. Traction is placed on the superior and inferior palpebral conjunctiva, the lacrimal puncta identified, and a mucocutaneous incision is made around the medial canthus temporal to the caruncle, 1 mm palpebral to and extending 2–3 mm temporal to the puncta (*A*). A second incision is made to isolate a triangular island of skin which contains the caruncle (*B*). The island of tissue is dissected free and discarded (*C*). The defect is closed in two layers: the conjunctiva is closed with interrupted 7-0 polygalactin 910 (Vicryl) with the knots buried (*D*, *E*), taking care not to include the puncta, and the skin apposed with simple interrupted sutures of 4-0 silk (*F*).

the cornea with accompanying pigment deposition and cellular infiltration (pinpoint gray infiltrates) (Figure 4-20).

Infiltration from the nasal limbus may occur in the latter stages of the disease.

Frequently accompanying the corneal changes are follicle formation, depigmentation, and thickening of the leading edge of the third eyelid. In some cases plasma cell infiltration of the third eyelids, with depigmentation, inflammation, and thickening, may be the sole presenting ocular sign, with little evidence of corneal pannus.

As the granulation tissue extends over the cornea and pigmentation becomes denser, visual impairment becomes progressively worse until the animal is blind.

DIAGNOSIS

On the basis of the characteristic bilateral clinical appearance of the corneal disease and breed incidence

DIFFERENTIAL DIAGNOSIS

Pigmentary keratitis due to other causes, including KCS, trichiasis, and lagophthalmos, is not always bilateral, does not have the classical distribution seen in pannus, and does not commonly affect the German Shepherd. The primary cause of the pigmentary keratitis may be obvious, such as an eyelid tumor, or is usually readily determined, as in using the Schirmer tear test in KCS.

PROGNOSIS AND TREATMENT

The owner of the dog must be warned that chronic superficial keratitis can be readily controlled but not cured. Treatment will be required for the rest of the dog's life, although there may be variation in the intensity of the treatment required for control. Corticosteroid therapy is usually successful in controlling the disease:

Initial aggressive treatment with a potent topical corticosteroid applied four times a day

Gradually decrease the frequency of application over six weeks until the preparation is being instilled once a day and eventually

---

The technique for lateral canthoplasty is similar in principle but facilitated by the absence of caruncle and puncta. Straight scissors are used to excise 3 mm of approximately a third the length of the superior and inferior temporal eyelids (*G*). Two-layer closure is performed as described above (*H, I*). From Peiffer RL Jr et al: Surgery of the canine and feline orbit, adnexa, and globe. Part II: Congenital abnormalities of the eyelid and cilia abnormalities. *Companion Animal Practice* 1:27–38, August 1987.

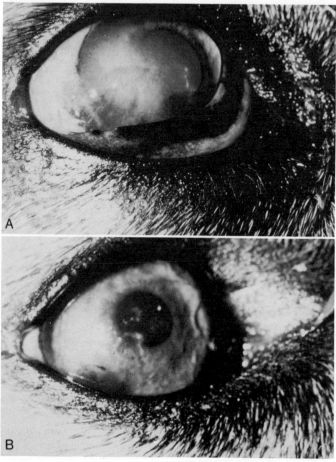

FIGURE 4-20. Early active chronic superficial keratitis (CSK pannus), right eye, in a three-year-old female German Shepherd. Note the temporal conjunctival pigment patch and corneal granulation and vascularization with a leading edge of infiltrate and edema (*A*). After four weeks of topical corticosteroid therapy, the condition is well controlled as indicated by absence of vascularization; a localized area of temporal corneal pigmentation remains (*B*). Secondary lipid dystrophy is present and not an uncommon finding in CSK. *C*, Advanced active pannus, left eye of a German Shepherd with more extensive pigmentary keratitis.

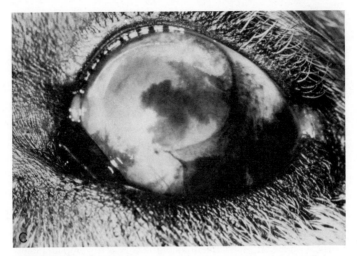

FIGURE 4–20, *Continued.*

on alternate days, as required to control the active process as indicated by infiltration, granulation, and vascularization.

If this intensive regimen of topical corticosteroids is not feasible due to poor owner compliance or the dog's temperament, or the response to topical therapy is poor, then a subconjunctival injection of a depot corticosteroid achieves dramatic improvement. Subconjunctival injections can be repeated once or twice at monthly intervals.

Subconjunctival injections of corticosteroid into the third eyelid will also help to reduce any accompanying plasma cell infiltration of this tissue.

Corticosteroids will dramatically reduce the vascularization of the cornea, but the pigment tends to remain (although it may thin over months). If pigmentation is causing visual impairment that is not improved by corticosteroids, then superficial keratectomy is indicated. After surgery, immediately commence treatment with topical antibiotics and corticosteroids to prevent corneal revascularization. This delays corneal epithelialization, and therefore the eye should be monitored closely for corneal complications.

Corneal Edema

Endothelial Dystrophies

Corneal endothelial dystrophies in veterinary practice are seen mainly in the dog, but occasionally also in the cat. They arise from degenerative changes in the corneal endothelial cells, whose normal function is to maintain stromal dehydration. There is a breed predisposition in the Boston Terrier, Dachshund, and Chihuahua, although the condition may be seen in middle-aged to old animals of any breed.

CLINICAL FINDINGS

Bilateral ocular disease in middle-aged to old dogs

Corneal edema begins as a blue or white cloudiness of the temporal cornea that progresses slowly until both corneas are totally opaque, usually within two to three years; less commonly, the process commences axially.

The condition is usually painless and the conjunctivae are not congested, but there may be very slight corneal vascularization towards the limbus as a secondary change.

Advanced cases may develop keratoconus (anterior conical protrusion of the edematous cornea).

Corneal bullae and subsequent ulcerations may develop and cause pain (blepharospasm and excessive lacrimation).

Vision is severely hampered in advanced cases due to corneal opacification.

Anterior Segment

Chronic Uveitis

Chronic uveitis is seen most commonly in the cat. Uveitis of long standing may be nongranulomatous (with a lymphocytic-plasmacytic cellular infiltrate) or granulomatous (with a cellular infiltration composed of macrophages, epithelioid histiocytes, and giant cells in addition to lymphocytes and plasma cells). The type of response is dependent on the nature of the initiating antigen. Keratic precipitates are the clinical hallmark of granulomatous uveitis.

ETIOLOGY

Idiopathic

Infectious: toxoplasmosis, oculomycoses (blastomycosis, histoplasmosis, coccidioidomycosis, cryptococcosis), tuberculosis, feline infectious peritonitis, feline leukemia-lymphosarcoma complex, leptospirosis, brucellosis, and leishmaniasis.

Lens-induced (leakage of lens material from cataractous lenses)

Autoimmune

Neoplastic: neoplasms (especially lymphosarcomas) metastatic or primary to the anterior uvea may mimic a nonresponsive uveitis

CLINICAL FINDINGS

Usually bilateral disease

The initial acute uveitis (blepharospasm, photophobia, excessive lacrimation, episcleral congestion, miotic pupil, sluggish pupillary light reflexes, aqueous flare, keratic precipitates, hypopyon, spongy swollen iris, and lowered intraocular pressure) gradually reduces in severity and progresses to a low-grade uveitis that occasionally flares up as acute bouts of ocular inflammation between periods of apparent quiescence.

In addition to the above-mentioned ocular findings in acute uveitis, chronic uveitis also manifests as:

Corneal edema and deep vascularization (deep keratitis)

Neovascularization and/or engorgement of the iris vasculature (particularly prominent in the cat)

Iris hyperpigmentation

Posterior synechiae (adhesions of the iris to the lens which distort the pupil). Neovascularization together with posterior synechiae formation may effectively obliterate the pupil due to the formation of a pseudomembrane.

Vision is impaired partially or totally by any of the above changes and the sequelae of chronic uveitis.

SEQUELAE

Cataract formation

Glaucoma (due to pupillary block by posterior synechiae, peripheral anterior synechiae, or obstruction of the iridocorneal angle by inflammatory cells and debris)

Retinal detachment (traction detachment due to formation and contraction of cyclitic membranes, or exudative detachment due to choroidal involvement)

Phthisis bulbi due to degeneration of the ciliary body and hypotony of the globe

DIAGNOSIS

On the basis of the history and clinical findings. Physical examination, hematology, serology, and blood biochemistry may be of use. Aqueous or vitreous paracentesis for cytology and culture may prove diagnostic in chronic infectious uveitis cases. Attempts to determine the etiology are frequently of no avail.

PROGNOSIS AND TREATMENT

Chronic uveitis responds poorly to treatment. Treat the primary disease if possible.

Corticosteroids help to relieve inflammation. Topical, subconjunctival, and also systemic steroids should be administered. Subconjunctival corticosteroids are useful in bouts of acute intraocular inflammation and may be utilized as long-term depot injections at monthly intervals.

Topical 1% atropine will relieve some of the pain of ciliary spasm and might help to break down posterior synechiae (this is rarely achieved with inactive adhesions); if the pupil is very miotic use 3 to 4% atropine and possibly also 2.5 to 10% phenylephrine over a short term.

Glaucoma

Cats

Primary glaucoma in the cat, although uncommon, does tend to present as a chronic progressive disease, unlike the acute congestive glaucomas seen in the dog.

ETIOLOGY

Primary glaucoma in the cat results from reduced aqueous outflow facility, possibly associated with abnormal drainage channels.

CLINICAL FINDINGS

Bilateral, occasionally unilateral disease with insidious onset in cats of various ages.

Older Siamese are predisposed.

Early cases show epiphora, anisocoria, some mild corneal edema, and mild episcleral congestion with a moderately elevated IOP (greater than 30 mm Hg).

Gonioscopy reveals open iridocorneal angles.

As the disease progresses, loss of vision and mydriasis become noticeable, with increasing intraocular pressure causing retinal degeneration (hyperreflective tapetal fundus), optic atrophy (sometimes with cupping of the disc), narrowing and eventual disappearance of retinal blood vessels, enlargement of the globe (hydrophthalmos) with exposure keratitis, and secondary lens luxation. The optic nerve and retina of the cat appear to be more resistant to elevated IOP than the dog, with some vision frequently persisting in the presence of advanced disease.

Iris atrophy may be seen.

DIAGNOSIS

On the basis of the history, ophthalmic findings and gonioscopy

DIFFERENTIAL DIAGNOSIS

Secondary glaucomas (due to intraocular inflammation, primary lens luxation, trauma, or neoplasia of the anterior uvea) are not usually bilateral. They present as a more acute onset glaucoma rather than the history of gradually increasing IOP and vision loss seen in primary glaucomas. Careful ophthalmic examination including gonioscopy will reveal the primary cause.

PROGNOSIS AND TREATMENT

Medical: control of IOP may be attempted using dichlorphenamide orally (25 mg BID) and topical 0.125% demecarium bromide (BID); however, response is usually unsatisfactory, and surgery offers the best chance for long-term maintenance of vision.

IOP should be monitored weekly. If IOP remains elevated with medical treatment, then surgery is indicated to save vision.

Surgical: corneoscleral trephination and peripheral iridectomy, cyclodialysis, iridencleisis, or an anterior chamber drainage tube are filtering procedures that may be performed. Vision often may be saved, and IOP can be controlled, allowing retention of the globe.

If the eye is grossly enlarged (buphthalmos), vision is irreversibly lost, and the animal is in pain, enucleation or evisceration with insertion of an intraocular prosthesis may be considered. Cyclocryotherapy is not as effective in the cat as in the dog. We believe intraocular gentamicin insertion to be contraindicated in cats because of occult preexisting or subsequently developing ocular sarcomas. Totally blind cats with bilateral hydrophthalmos frequently adapt amazingly well; if the animal is unable to cope with the disability, euthanasia may be preferable.

Dogs

Primary open-angle glaucoma in the dog is an uncommon condition resulting in progressive visual impairment due to a slow rise in intraocular pressure. This is caused by increased resistance to aqueous filtration in the drainage channels, resulting in decreased outflow facility. The disease is inherited as an autosomal recessive trait in the Beagle, but can also occur in other breeds, including Toy and Miniature Poodles.

CLINICAL FINDINGS

Bilateral disease (in Beagles from 1 to 3 years of age)
Initially there is slight mydriasis and mild episcleral congestion. IOP at this stage is about 35 to 45 mm Hg (normal 15 to 30 mm Hg).

Initially gonioscopy reveals an open iridocorneal angle.

Over time the iridocorneal angle steadily becomes narrower and closes.

Gonioscopy in moderately advanced cases reveals some areas where the iridocorneal angle is open and some where it is closed.

As IOP continues to rise, vision gradually deteriorates with generalized retinal degeneration (hyperreflective tapetal fundus), optic disk cupping, optic atrophy, loss of retinal vasculature, and eventually globe enlargement with consequent exposure keratopathy.

An acute rise in IOP often results from secondary lens luxation (with subsequent cataract formation) causing vitreolental pupillary block. Such eyes show signs typical of acute congestive glaucoma (mydriasis, episcleral congestion, corneal edema, pain, blepharospasm, and excessive lacrimation).

DIAGNOSIS

The findings of ophthalmic examination, including gonioscopy and tonometry of both eyes

Breed incidence

PROGNOSIS AND TREATMENT

If gonioscopy reveals an open iridocorneal angle (early stage), there is usually a good response to medical treatment of topical 0.25% demecarium bromide (BID) and oral dichlorphenamide (10 mg/kg BID). The IOP should be monitored initially at weekly intervals to ensure the efficacy of the treatment regimen. If the iridocorneal angle is narrowed and the lens subluxated (moderately advanced stage), then medical treatment as above may be successful in controlling IOP, but usually only temporally. If IOP cannot be controlled medically, then a surgical filtering procedure is indicated. The prognosis is reasonable if the disease is not advanced and the retina and optic nerve are still somewhat functional. Irreversibly blind globes are managed by one of the procedures available to obtain cosmesis.

Cataracts

Cataract is a nonspecific disease that results in opacification of the lens fibers or capsule. Cataracts may be characterized clinically according to stage of development, location within the lens, age of the animal at the time of development, and etiology.

The stages of development of a cataract include the initial opacity and, if the cataract is progressive, subsequent degeneration of the lens. The stages of development are incipient, immature, mature, and hypermature.

Incipient. Focal opacification of the lens or its capsule. The animal can still see well. This stage may or may not be progressive.

Immature. Opacity is more or less diffuse, although there may be areas of variable density. The fundic reflex is still present and vision may or may not be impaired. Mature lens opacification is total and dense, with absence of the fundic reflex. Visual function is significantly impaired. Mature cataractous lenses may become hydrated and increase in size (intumescence). Cataract surgery is recommended at this stage.

Hypermature. Lens protein liquefies and may leak through the capsule. If leakage is extensive with significant resorption of protein, the lens capsule becomes wrinkled or dimpled, initially at the equator. The nucleus, which is insoluble albuminoid protein, may migrate inferiorly within the lens capsule to form a Morgagnian cataract. Uveitis may result from leakage of lens protein. The fundic reflex may be present peripherally, and the animal may see if resorption is extensive.

Location is an aid in defining etiology, and cataracts may be capsular, subcapsular, cortical, or nuclear. These are further described as axial or equatorial, anterior or posterior, and according to the position of the hands on a clock (e.g., three o'clock position).

Age of the animal when the cataract first appears may be used to classify the cataract as one of the following:

Congenital. The cataract is present at birth. Congenital cataracts may be inherited or noninherited.

Developmental. An inherited bilateral cataract that occurs after birth, usually in young animals, but in such breeds as the American Cocker Spaniel, Miniature Poodle, and Boston Terrier may not appear until later in life.

Senile. Occurring in aged animals, preceded or accompanied by nuclear sclerosis.

Etiology may be difficult to determine. Cataracts may occur secondary to ocular diseases, including uveitis, retinal degeneration, and glaucoma; in association with systemic metabolic disease, including diabetes mellitus and Cushing's disease; secondary to blunt or penetrating trauma; or they may represent a congenital developmental disorder. The majority of canine cataracts are primary inherited cataracts. Cataracts are much less common in the cat and usually are secondary to trauma and/or uveitis.

Hereditary Cataract

Primary Hereditary Cataracts. Cataracts not associated with any other ocular or systemic disease are the most common type of canine cataract. Hereditary cataracts are bilateral with a distinct breed incidence and usually have a typical appearance and age of onset: they may be congenital or not manifest until much later in life. Clinical features of hereditary cataracts are summarized in Table 4–2.

PROGNOSIS AND TREATMENT

Cataracts are a surgical disease; no reliable topical, systemic, or intraocular medication prevents progression or induces resorption.

Extracapsular lens extraction is routinely performed for the majority of cataract extractions; due to the strong hyaloideocapsular ligament, intracapsular extraction almost invariably results in disruption of the hyaloid membrane with increased incidence of vitreous presentation and associated complications, including corneal edema, glaucoma, and retinal detachment. With the extracapsular technique, the posterior lens capsule and vitreous face are not disturbed.

The objective of cataract surgery is to restore functional vision. Because of the ability of dogs and cats to adjust and compensate for incomplete lens opacity or monocular blindness, functional vision is not significantly impaired until bilateral cataracts approach maturity. The owner of the pet is usually the best judge of when surgery should be contemplated. When the animal is constantly bumping into objects and is unable to maintain its normal lifestyle and personality, cataract extraction should be considered.

Establishing the integrity of the retina and the central visual pathways is of prime importance. Both client and surgeon are discouraged when a technically successful procedure fails to restore vision because of concurrent disease of the retina or optic nerve. To evaluate the neural visual components, history, ophthalmoscopy, visual function tests, and electrophysiology should be used in combination.

Inherited retinal degeneration is increasing in incidence and is the primary reason for failure in technically successful cataract surgery. Owing to mechanisms that are poorly understood, animals with inherited or inflammatory retinal degeneration are likely to develop associated cataracts. The problem is complicated by the fact that breeds with a high incidence of inherited retinal degeneration (e.g., the Miniature and Toy Poodles and the Irish Setter) also have primary genetic cataracts unassociated with retinal disease.

Evaluating pupillary responses is unreliable as a sole method of assessing peripheral and central visual potential. The majority of cataract patients should demonstrate complete brisk, direct, and consensual responses to a bright focal light source in a darkened room in the presence of even the densest cataract. With some variability, these responses persist in the presence of well-advanced retinal degeneration. The ganglion cell nerve fibers that mediate this reflex are distinct from the visual fibers that extend to the lateral geniculate body and thus provide no information as to the status of the optic radiation and visual cortex. Iris atrophy is not infrequently observed in Miniature and Toy Poodles, and lesions involving the third cranial nerve may also result in an absence of pupillary reflexes in the presence of intact visual components. Thus, although normal pupillary reflexes are always reassuring, they provide minimal definitive information.

History is helpful in proportion to the owner's awareness of changes in the animal's appearance and behavior. Without exception, visual and ophthalmoscopic changes in inherited retinal degeneration always precede associated cataract development. Thus, a reliable history that visual impairment accompanied or followed rather than preceded noticeable cataract development speaks in favor of an intact visual system. If inherited retinal degeneration is present, a history of initial nyctalopia (night blindness) may be elicited. Critical ophthalmoscopy performed while the cataracts are still immature, rather than waiting until the fundus cannot be critically examined, is of benefit to all involved. Ophthalmoscopy prior to maturity of the cataract approaches one hundred percent reliability. The rare dog with genetic tendencies to develop both retinal degeneration and primary cataracts will provide an occasional disappointment if the retinal degeneration develops subsequent to the primary cataract.

Testing the ability to negotiate an obstacle course under photopic and scotopic conditions may be of value in cases in which fundus reflex can be obtained, although lens changes prohibit critical fundic examination. As a general rule, if a fundic reflex can be obtained, some vision should be present and should change minimally with alterations in ambient light if the retina is healthy.

Electrophysiology provides the most reliable criteria for critical evaluation. Ideally, an electroretinogram should be performed in all patients with cataracts; in breeds predisposed to inherited retinal degeneration, electroretinography is a prerequisite to cataract surgery.

The surgeon who attempts cataract surgery without an electroretinogram will have fewer successes than a surgeon who utilizes the test. If the history, pupillary responses, or neurologic findings suggest the possibility of a defect in the central visual system, evaluation of visually evoked response may be considered in addition to electroretinography. Ultrasonography may be of value in the presurgical detection of retinal detachment.

A large percentage of young dogs (between one and three years) with inherited developmental cataracts (seen most frequently in the Afghan Hound, American Cocker Spaniel, Irish Setter, and Miniature and Toy Poodle) undergo a spontaneous resorption of their cataracts. The resorption of feline cataracts follows a similar pattern. Active resorption, indicated by mild

TABLE 4-2. Clinical Features of Inherited Canine Cataracts

BREED	MODE OF GENETIC TRANSMISSION	AGE OF ONSET	CHARACTERISTIC EARLY APPEARANCE	BIOLOGIC BEHAVIOR
American Cocker Spaniel (type 1)		Congenital	Nuclear and cortical	Slowly progressive
Boston Bull Terrier (type 1)	Recessive	Congenital–4 months	Nuclear and cortical	Slowly progressive; mature by 2 years
German Shepherd	Recessive	Congenital–2–3 months	Posterior cortical/suture line vacuoles; extension to nucleus and cortex	Progressive; equatorial cortex spared
Golden Retriever (type 1)		Congenital	Nuclear and cortical	Slowly progressive
Miniature Schnauzer	Recessive	Congenital–4 months	Nuclear and cortical	Slowly progressive; mature by 2 years
Old English Sheepdog		Congenital–2 years	Nuclear and cortical	Progressive
Staffordshire Bull Terrier	Recessive	Congenital–4 months	Nuclear and cortical	Slowly progressive; mature by 2 years
Welsh Springer Spaniel	Recessive	Congenital–4 months	Cortical	Progressive; mature by 1.5–2 years
Beagle	Dominant	4 months	Posterior axial opacities	Nonprogressive
Afghan Hound	Recessive	4 mos–2 yrs	Equatorial vacuoles	Rapidly progressive
Irish Setter	Recessive	4 mos–2 yrs	Cortical	Rapidly progressive
Siberian Husky	Recessive	6 mos–2 yrs	Posterior axial subcapsular opacity ± cortical vacuoles	Very slowly progressive

Breed	Inheritance	Location/Type	Age	Progression
Standard Poodle	Recessive	Equatorial	Congenital–2 years	Progressive; mature by 1–3 years
Golden Retriever (type 2)		Axial posterior subcapsular triangular opacity	9–18 mos	Usually nonprogressive
Labrador Retriever		Axial posterior subcapsular triangular opacity	9–18 mos	Usually nonprogressive
Large Munsterlander		Axial posterior subcapsular triangular opacity	9–18 mos	Usually nonprogressive
Belgian Sheepdog		Axial posterior subcapsular triangular opacity	9–18 mos	Usually progressive
Chesapeake Bay Retriever	Dominant with incomplete penetrance	Posterior subcapsular, axial or equatorial	variable	Slowly progressive
American Cocker Spaniel	Recessive	cortical	6 mos–8 yrs	Often asymmetric; stable or slowly progressive for months to years, then rapid progression to maturity
Miniature and Toy Poodles	Recessive	cortical	2–10 years	Progressive
Boston Bull Terrier (type 2)		Radiating cuneiform (wedgelike) cortical opacities	4–12 years	Very slowly progressive

lens-induced uveitis and an irregular lens capsule, is an indication for temporization. Although these liquefied cataracts may be aspirated, approximately thirty percent resorb to the extent that cataract surgery is unnecessary. These animals should be managed with topical application of 1.0% atropine sulfate to enhance peripheral vision and corticosteroids to temper the uveitis. Such cases should be examined monthly, and cataract surgery should be recommended only when active resorption has subsided without restoration of visual function.

Cataract surgery is an elective procedure; thorough multisystem evaluation should be performed prior to surgery. Concurrent related disease (diabetes mellitus or Cushing's disease) or unrelated disease (renal decompensation or heartworm disease) should be identified and adequately controlled. In older patients with systemic disease who have adjusted reasonably well to their visual impairment, the risk of complications of anesthesia should be weighed against the benefits of restoring vision.

Unilateral or bilateral surgery may be performed, either at one or two sittings, based upon the wishes of the client and the visual requirements of the patient. Older house pets gain adequate functional vision with unilateral surgery; younger, more active animals and obedience or hunting dogs may benefit greatly from bilateral cataract extraction.

Current trends suggest that the use of phacoemulsification and/or phacofragmentation and the insertion of an artificial lens will soon be routine in veterinary cataract surgery. Ultrasonic disruption of cataractous lens material followed by its aspiration presents a reasonable alternative to the extracapsular techniques described above; however, the expense and sophistication of the instrumentation limits its routine use to institutions or practices that perform large volumes of cataract surgery. Success rates will most likely prove to be similar to, if not superior to, that of manual "open-sky" extraction, primarily because the entire procedure is performed within a formed anterior chamber, which tends to minimize iris exudation and constriction.

The use of intraocular plastic lenses has achieved widespread acceptance in human ophthalmology. We have had excellent results with the use of a posterior chamber intraocular lens specifically designed for the canine eye in terms of size and refractive power (30 diopters). Not only does the implant markedly improve visual function following surgery but also it minimizes the complications of posterior synechiae between iris and lens capsule that are commonly encountered utilizing the standard techniques. The implant must be inserted in a formed chamber filled with viscoelastic material such as hyaluronic acid. The incidence of lens-related complications is low, and we strongly feel that the benefits of increased vision and fewer adhesions outweigh the additional expense and slightly increased risk factors in those patients whose owners are willing to opt for intraocular lens insertion.

The procedure for cataract removal, when performed with appropriate preoperative treatment and instrumentation, is not difficult and optimal success rates approach ninety percent. The incidence of intraoperative or postoperative complications, however, is high compared to that for other procedures, and these complications frequently have disastrous effects on the outcome of the surgery. The surgeon's experience and understanding of ocular anatomy, physiology, and pathology facilitate the recognition and management of complications. With regard to technical refinement, the routine use of microsurgical techniques and anterior vitrectomy also significantly improves results. For those reasons we believe that the operation is best performed by a specialist.

Secondary Hereditary Cataracts

These cataracts are associated with other primary hereditary ocular diseases, including progressive retinal atrophy, retinal dysplasia, microphthalmos with multiple congenital ocular anomalies, and lens luxation.

Several breeds of dog show cataract formation associated with recessively inherited, generalized PRA. In practice these are most commonly encountered in the Miniature and Toy Poodles and the English Cocker Spaniel. Secondary cataracts develop after ophthalmoscopic signs of PRA become apparent. History reveals that visual problems, especially nyctalopia (night blindness), developed before the onset of cataractous changes. These cataracts are bilateral and are usually seen in middle-aged dogs. The posterior axial and equatorial cortex of the lens is affected first with vacuoles spreading centrally; the cataracts are progressive over several months to years. Pupillary light reflexes tend to be sluggish but may be normal even in the presence of significant clinical disease. Ophthalmoscopy through areas of immature cataract may reveal tapetal fundus hyperreflectivity typical of PRA; however, if the cataracts are total, electroretinography should be considered as the most reliable means to assess retinal function prior to cataract surgery.

Cataracts associated with central PRA (possibly irregular dominant inheritance) are far less common than those associated with generalized PRA but may still occur. For example, Labrador Retrievers with central PRA (retinal pigment epithelial dystrophy) may develop cortical cataracts that are slowly progressive. Ophthalmoscopy will usually reveal fundus changes typical of central PRA (pigmentary disturbance and later hyperreflectivity over the tapetal fundus).

If PRA is present, then the cataractous lenses should not be removed unless they dislocate and threaten loss of the eye due to secondary glaucoma.

Cortical cataracts may be seen secondary to total retinal dysplasia (retinal nonattachment or detachment), which is inherited as an autosomal recessive trait in the Labrador Retriever, English Springer Spaniel, and Sealyham and Bedlington Terriers. In the English Springer Spaniel in particular, retinal detachment and secondary cataract formation may be unilateral; therefore, check the other eye for evidence of retinal folds and areas of involvement.

Hereditary congenital cataracts associated with multiple ocular defects are also seen in several breeds of dog. They are usually bilateral and similar in the two eyes. In the Miniature Schnauzer, microphthalmos with mainly nuclear cataract and posterior lenticonus is inherited as a recessive condition. Microphakia and nystagmus may also be present. The nuclear cataracts rarely progress, although any cortical extensions may progress slowly.

Microphthalmos, nuclear cataract (sometimes with cortical extensions), posterior lenticonus, and iris hypoplasia are seen in the Cavalier King Charles Spaniel; genetics have not been defined. The Old English Sheepdog, by possible autosomal recessive inheritance, demonstrates microphthalmos, nuclear and/or cortical cataract, retinal dysplasia, and anisocoria.

The English Cocker Spaniel has a condition of microphthalmos, nuclear and/or cortical cataract, anterior lenticonus, persistent pupillary membranes, retinal dysplasia, and nystagmus; genetics have not been defined.

Similar congenital cataracts associated with other ocular anomalies have also been reported in the West Highland White Terrier, Beagle, and Golden Retriever breeds.

TREATMENT

If puppies are presented with extensive cataracts and severe accompanying ocular defects (e.g., severe microphthalmos or extensive persistent pupillary membranes), then euthanasia should be considered. Puppies with some visual impairment due mainly to nuclear cataracts can be allowed to mature. Normal cortical lens fibers are laid down around the lens so the nuclear cataract becomes relatively smaller and vision improves. Nuclear cataracts are rarely progressive. Mydriatic eyedrops (1% atropine applied 2 to 3 times per week) can also help to extend these dogs' visual fields.

If the degree of microphthalmos and other anomalies is not severe but the cataract is extensive (nuclear and cortical) or total, then cataract extraction can be considered. However, the prognosis in these individuals should be more guarded due to other accompanying defects and increased incidence of complications.

Cataract surgery in young animals must be performed early in life to permit proper development of the central visual system.

Developmental Cataracts

Developmental cataracts manifest later in life. They include the primary hereditary cataracts mentioned earlier. Other less common causes of developmental cataracts include trauma, dietary deficiencies, toxic agents, radiation, metabolic disturbances, and intraocular inflammation.

Senile Cataracts

Senile cataracts develop in older dogs and cats because of age-related degenerative changes in the lens. They occur usually as wedge-shaped cortical opacities, progress slowly, and are rarely of clinical significance (Figure 4–21).

Nuclear sclerosis should not be confused with true cataractous changes in the lens. Nuclear sclerosis is a very common, normal, age-related physiological change within the lens and is seen in most older dogs and very old cats. It results from compression and hardening of the nuclear fibers at the center of the lens, which alters their refractive properties. Nuclear sclerosis imparts a slightly cloudy or bluish appearance to the pupil, but it does not impair vision. The margins of the central zone of sclerosis are distinct, and a fundus reflex is obtainable through it. Ophthalmoscopy of the fundus is possible through the sclerotic lens but not through a true cataract.

Traumatic Cataracts

Penetrating injuries from shotgun pellets, thorns, and cat claws that penetrate the anterior lens capsule and disrupt lens fibers in the anterior cortex may cause traumatic cataracts. If the degree of disruption of lens fibers is minimal, then the cataract may not progress, but severe disruption results in rapidly progressive cataractous changes. Blunt injuries and blows to the globe as in road traffic accidents may result in cataracts either by tearing the anterior lens capsule, with cortical cataract formation, or by adversely affecting the lens in the presence of an intact capsule.

CLINICAL FINDINGS

Usually unilateral

Evidence of trauma to the eye is often apparent (conjunctival hemorrhage and/or bruising, corneal laceration and/or edema).

Slitlamp biomicroscopy may be required to appreciate capsular damage caused by penetrating injuries.

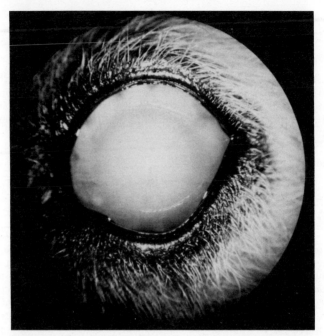

FIGURE 4-21. Senile cataract in a twelve-year-old female Miniature Poodle, left eye. Nuclear sclerosis has progressed to cataract, with absence of fundus reflex. The cortex is characterized by cuneiform opacities.

Frequently leakage of lens material through the damaged lens capsule elicits anterior uveitis and even severe endophthalmitis may ensue (ocular pain, excessive lacrimation, photophobia, blepharospasm, episcleral congestion, lowered intraocular pressure, aqueous flare and/or hypopyon, formation of anterior or posterior synechiae, and sometimes leading to glaucoma and phthisis bulbi).

DIAGNOSIS

On the basis of the history and findings of ophthalmic examination A foreign body may be identified on x-ray.

TREATMENT

Therapy should be directed toward the control of the lens-induced uveitis with topical 1% atropine repeated frequently, topical and systemic corticosteroids, and systemic antibiotic cover. Surgical extraction of the lens may be required if there is gross leakage of lens material before this condition results in uncontrollable intraocular inflammation.

Dietary-Deficiency Cataracts

Deficiencies of several amino acids and vitamin B complex have been shown to produce cataracts in experimental animals. This is rarely encountered in veterinary practice except in young animals reared on inadequately fortified milk substitutes.

Toxic Cataracts

Toxic cataracts result from numerous chemical agents (naphthalene, dinitrophenol, thallium, selenium) and some therapeutic drugs, (corticosteroids, contraceptives, insulin, chlorpromazine, and echothiophate). Generally, these cases are rare in practice.

Cataracts Secondary to Inflammation

Uveitis may result in cataract formation. These cataracts arise because of alterations in the composition of the aqueous and/or vitreous on which the lens relies for its nutrition and removal of waste products.

Cataracts secondary to uveitis also result from posterior synechiae in which inflamed iris adheres to the anterior lens capsule, affects its permeability, and causes opacification of the capsule and often subcapsular cortical cataract.

CLINICAL FINDINGS

Total or partial opacification of the lens

Unilateral; if bilateral, then the cataracts tend to be asymmetrical

Evidence of past episodes of uveitis are often present, including posterior synechiae, pigment or inflammatory debris on the anterior lens capsule, thickening and hyperpigmentation of the iris, and precipitates on the posterior surface of the cornea.

If the fundus can be visualized, there may be evidence of chorioretinitis and vitreous syneresis.

DIAGNOSIS

On the basis of the history of ocular inflammation and/or pain and the findings of ophthalmic examination

TREATMENT AND PROGNOSIS

Cataract severity and progression tend to be roughly proportional to the duration and severity of the uveitis. Focal opacification will not progress if inflammation is localized and will require no surgical treatment if vision is not markedly impaired. Mature cataracts may be successfully removed with a guarded prognosis; incidence of intra- and postoperative complications is higher in these patients. Extensive chorioretinitis or retinal detachment may be obscured by a total cataract so that even if surgical extraction of the cataractous lens is successful, vision is very poor or absent. Electroretinography and ultrasonography are recommended in those cases in which surgery is anticipated.

Diabetic Cataracts

Cataracts develop in most dogs and some cats suffering from diabetes mellitus. In this disease, because of altered glucose metabolism, sorbitol accumulates within the lens and alters its osmotic potential. Cataract formation then results from water influx and breakdown of lens fibers.

CLINICAL FINDINGS

Bilateral, symmetrical, rapidly developing cataracts (sometimes within days)

The earliest changes are seen as vacuoles in the equatorial cortex (mydriasis is required in order to appreciate this).

Classical mature diabetic cataracts exhibit *water-clefts*, linear breaks within the cataractous lens, usually along the suture lines.

DIAGNOSIS

Cataracts in a breed other than those commonly affected by hereditary cataracts (Miniature Poodle, American Cocker Spaniel, and Boston Terrier) should raise suspicion

History of polyphagia and polydipsia with rapid-onset bilateral cataracts

Urine and blood biochemistry to confirm that diabetes mellitus is the primary metabolic disturbance

PROGNOSIS AND TREATMENT

Ensure that the diabetes mellitus is controlled first! Surgical extraction of the cataracts usually results in restoration of vision.

Diabetic retinopathy, though rarely seen, does occur in the dog, but unlike man it is usually relatively mild, with microaneurysms and minor retinal hemorrhages. It occurs in chronic cases of diabetes mellitus and may be seen ophthalmoscopically after successful cataract extraction.

Vitreous

Vitritis and vitreous hemorrhage may occasionally present as chronic visual loss but are more often of acute onset and are described in detail elsewhere.

Retina and Choroid

Inherited retinal degenerations are frequently responsible for chronic loss of vision in the dog and cat. Commonly referred to as *progressive retinal atrophy* (PRA), these retinal dystrophies and degenerations exhibit a distinct breed and age incidence. These conditions in the dog may be grouped into two types: generalized PRA (which is by far the most common) and central PRA.

Generalized PRA

Generalized PRA consists of a group of inherited retinal disorders, all of which show autosomal recessive inheritance and are primarily diseases of the photoreceptors (the inner retinal layers may degenerate as a secondary phenomenon). At least three distinct diseases fall within the broad classification of generalized PRA: rod-cone dysplasia, rod dysplasia, and progressive rod-cone dysplasia.

Rod-cone Dysplasia

Rod-cone dysplasia is an early-onset retinal dystrophy characterized by retarded differentiation of the rod and cone photoreceptors, followed by their subsequent degeneration. It has been demonstrated biochemically in two breeds that the photoreceptors show abnormal cyclic nucleotide metabolism, accumulating toxic levels of cyclic guanosine monophosphate (cGMP). This is due to deficient activity of the enzyme cGMP-phosphodiesterase.

BREED INCIDENCE

Irish Setter, Collie, and perhaps the Norwegian Elkhound and Miniature Long-haired Dachshund

CLINICAL FINDINGS

Initial night blindness (nyctalopia) followed by progressive, slow, and relentless loss of daytime vision; the dog may be afraid of dark conditions.

Observant owners may notice tunnel vision as the peripheral visual field is reduced; the dog may see only objects directly in front of it, and it will tend to lose sight of moving objects, such as a thrown ball, as they move out of its central gaze.

Age of onset is very young, 6 to 12 weeks.

Total blindness is apparent by 1 to 2 years

Ophthalmoscopy at 3 to 4 months reveals bilaterally symmetrical hyperreflectivity over the tapetal fundus, starting at the periphery and spreading centrally (Figure 4-22,A).

Following this, there is narrowing of retinal blood vessels and patchy depigmentation of the nontapetal fundus

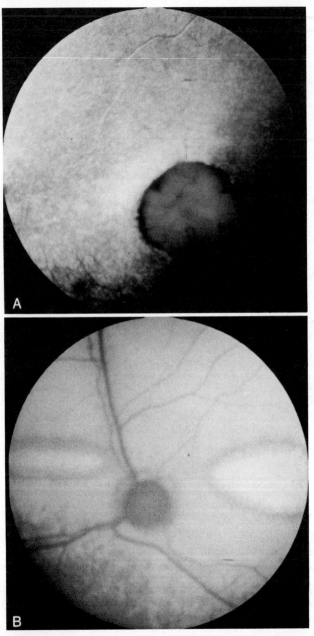

FIGURE 4-22. *See legend on the opposite page.*

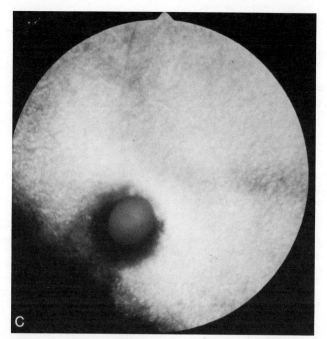

FIGURE 4–22. Retinal atrophy. *A,* Inherited progressive retinal atrophy in a Japanese Akita. The ophthalmoscopic triad of retinal vasculature attenuation, tapetal hyperreflectivity, and optic atrophy are evident. *B,* Feline central retinal degeneration. Linear zones of hyperreflectivity are seen both nasal and temporal to the optic disk. *C,* Nutritional retinal atrophy in a young domestic shorthair cat fed dog food exclusively.

Optic disk atrophy follows, the disk appearing pale.
Secondary cataracts frequently develop as a late finding.

DIAGNOSIS

Breed of dog, with characteristic history of visual loss and age of onset

Bilaterally symmetrical progressive ophthalmoscopic degenerative changes

Electroretinography in very young puppies (4 to 6 weeks) can detect rod-cone dysplasia. The ERG is grossly abnormal with absent rod responses and reduced cone function.

TREATMENT

None. Affected puppies are probably best euthanized. Because the visual loss is slowly progressive, however, affected dogs can adapt quite well to their disability and show remarkable confidence as long as they are kept in a familiar environment.

Rod Dysplasia

This disease is characterized by defective development of the rod photoreceptors with secondary degeneration of the cones.

BREED INCIDENCE

Norwegian Elkhound

CLINICAL FINDINGS

Initial nyctalopia may be detected as early as 2 to 3 months of age (more usually noticed at 6 to 12 months) with normal day vision.

Vision deteriorates progressively to total blindness by 3 to 6 years

Ophthalmoscopic changes become apparent by 6 to 12 months of age, beginning with a brown, granular discoloration of the tapetal fundus and progressing to peripheral tapetal hyperreflectivity and retinal vessel attenuation.

Later the hyperreflectivity becomes generalized over the tapetal fundus, the retinal blood vessels disappear, patchy depigmentation is apparent in the nontapetal fundus, and the optic disk becomes atrophic.

DIAGNOSIS

Breed of dog, age of onset of progressive visual loss, and bilaterally symmetrical ophthalmoscopic findings

ERGs of young affected Norwegian Elkhounds (as early as 6 weeks) show absent rod function but retained cone function.

TREATMENT

As for rod-cone dysplasia

Progressive Rod-Cone Degeneration

This late-onset disease is an *abiotrophy*, that is, the photoreceptors show normal development, but degenerate in later years. Affected photoreceptors show reduced turnover rates of outer segments. Rods degenerate faster than cones.

BREED INCIDENCE

Toy and Miniature Poodles, Tibetan Terrier, and the English Cocker Spaniel.

CLINICAL FINDINGS

Night blindness is the first detectable sign, between 2 and 4 years of age in Poodles, 1 and 2 years in the Tibetan Terrier, and 2 and 3 years in English Cocker Spaniels.

Day blindness follows, with progression to total blindness by 5 to 8 years of age.

Pupillary light reflexes are sluggish at this late stage.

Ophthalmoscopic changes are apparent as hyperreflectivity of the peripheral tapetal fundus, which spreads centrally. Ophthalmoscopic changes are apparent before owners notice visual impairment.

Accompanying the hyperreflectivity is retinal blood vessel narrowing.

Later there is patchy depigmentation of the nontapetal fundus and optic disk pallor (optic atrophy).

Secondary cataract formation is frequently, if not invariably, observed over several months to years after the retinal degeneration. Cataractous changes usually begin in the posterior cortex of the lens.

DIAGNOSIS

History of night blindness followed by progressive loss of vision

Breed and age incidence and bilaterally symmetrical ophthalmoscopic changes.

ERGs of early affected animals show responses of reduced amplitude and prolonged implicit times.

TREATMENT

None effective generalized PRA has also been reported to occur in other breeds, including the Labrador Retriever, English Springer Spaniel, Tibetan Spaniel, Cardigan Welsh Corgi, Cairn Terrier, Samoyed, Miniature Schnauzer, and Japanese Akita, as well as mixed-breed animals.

Because generalized PRA is inherited as an autosomal recessive disease, affected dogs, both of their parents (which are at least carriers), and any offspring should not be used for future breeding. Carriers can be detected by test-mating with an affected dog. Electroretinography may be used in the early detection of affected dogs, especially in the rod-cone dysplasias.

Central PRA

Central PRA is a retinal pigment epithelial dystrophy. Degeneration of the photoreceptors and other retinal layers occurs secondary to the failure of the retinal pigment epithelium to phagocytose shed outer segment disks. The disease causes an initial central visual loss, reflecting the name of the disease.

BREED INCIDENCE

Labrador Retriever (possible autosomal dominant inheritance with incomplete penetrance), Golden Retriever, Border Collie, Rough Collie, Smooth Collie, Shetland Sheepdog, English Springer Spaniel, and Cardigan Corgi (mode of inheritance unknown), and Briard (autosomal recessive inheritance).

CLINICAL FINDINGS

Variable age of onset: 1 to 6 years of age and even later in Briards

Vision loss is first apparent in daylight, particularly in those dogs used for hunting. Moving objects are readily seen, but stationary objects directly in front of the animal are often missed. Vision improves at night. When called, the dog may look at the owner with its head turned slightly to one side, as the animal is using its more functional peripheral retina.

Visual loss is slowly progressive but not usually to total blindness. Some peripheral vision tends to be preserved even in old dogs.

Pupillary light reflexes become sluggish in older affected dogs.

Ophthalmoscopy shows initial pigmentary disturbance in the central tapetal fundus superior temporal to the optic disk (temporal peripheral tapetal fundus in the Briard). This is characterized by multiple foci of brown pigment (lipopigment). Ophthalmoscopic changes occur prior to evidence of visual impairment. Reducing the light intensity of the ophthalmoscope (or even using a green filter) will help to detect the early subtle pigmentary changes.

Pigment foci become more numerous and appear to coalesce, eventually fading with advancing disease.

Hyperreflectivity of the tapetal fundus also becomes evident.

Late changes are retinal blood vessel attenuation, mottled depigmentation of the nontapetal fundus, and optic atrophy.

Secondary cataracts sometimes occur.

DIAGNOSIS

Breed incidence
History of characteristic visual loss
Bilaterally symmetrical ophthalmoscopic changes

TREATMENT

No treatment will cure the disease, although occasional use of a topical mydriatic (1% atropine applied every 2 to 3 days) may improve vision. Affected dogs usually cope well and adapt to their gradual loss of sight as long as they are in a familiar environment.

Avoid breeding from affected animals, their parents, and any progeny.

Hemeralopia

Hemeralopia (day blindness) is an uncommon hereditary disease in the dog caused by a partial or total failure in development of cone photoreceptors with their subsequent degeneration or by a cone degeneration per se. This results, eventually, in a totally rod photoreceptor retina.

BREED INCIDENCE

Alaskan Malamute (autosomal recessive inheritance) and possibly the Miniature Poodle and German Shepherd

CLINICAL FINDINGS

History of day blindness with improved vision in poor light
Affected dogs are noticed between 2 and 6 months of age.
These dogs repeatedly collide with objects in bright light, whereas in dim light (after several minutes of adaptation) they are able to negotiate these objects. Day blindness becomes progressively worse.
Ophthalmoscopy reveals no abnormalities.
Pupillary light reflexes are normal.

DIAGNOSIS

Breed incidence
Characteristic visual loss and behavior
Normal fundus on ophthalmoscopy
ERG reveals normal rod function and abnormal cone function

DIFFERENTIAL DIAGNOSIS

Central PRA: dogs may also show poor vision in daylight and improved vision at night. Central PRA has a different breed incidence (retrievers, collies, and the Briard) and characteristic progressive fundus changes (pigment foci, etc.).

TREATMENT

None

Inherited Retinal Degeneration in the Cat

This condition is not as common as in the dog, but there are several reports of proven inherited retinal dystrophies in the cat, including autosomal, recessively inherited early-onset retinal degeneration in Persian kittens and autosomal, dominantly inherited early-onset retinal degeneration in litters of cats of mixed breeding (rod-cone dysplasia).

In both cases, kittens showed marked visual impairment at a few weeks of age.
Vision was rapidly lost to total blindness.
Ophthalmoscopy revealed bilaterally symmetrical tapetal fundus hyperreflectivity and retinal vessel attenuation progressing to

an advanced atrophic appearance with disappearance of the retinal vasculature.

ERGs were markedly subnormal.

The Abyssinian breed of cat suffers from two distinct types of inherited retinal dystrophy: An early-onset rod-cone dysplasia and a late-onset rod-cone degeneration.

Early-Onset Rod-Cone Dysplasia Inherited as an Autosomal Dominant Trait

Early-onset, autosomal dominantly inherited rod-cone dysplasia in Abyssinian cats is similar to PRA in the Irish Setter and also associated with abnormal retinal cyclic nucleotide metabolism. This disease does not appear to be a field problem.

CLINICAL FINDINGS

Affected kittens show dilated pupils and sluggish pupillary light reflexes at 2 to 3 weeks of age.

Nystagmus develops at 4 to 6 weeks.

Vision is present although impaired. Affected animals show progressive visual loss but retain light perception.

Bilaterally symmetrical ophthalmoscopic changes begin in the area centralis with tapetal fundus hyperreflectivity at 8 to 12 weeks of age.

Hyperreflectivity spreads and is followed by attenuation of the retinal blood vessels.

Late changes are patchy depigmentation of the nontapetal fundus and focal tapetal degeneration in the area centralis in some cats.

The ERG is absent or grossly subnormal.

Late-Onset Rod-Cone Degeneration Inherited as an Autosomal Recessive Trait

This is a common problem in European Abyssinian cats and is similar to PRA in the Miniature Poodle.

CLINICAL FINDINGS

Cats become affected at 1.5 to 2 years of age.

There is progression to total blindness over 2 to 3 years.

Ophthalmoscopy reveals bilaterally symmetrical changes beginning with altered reflectivity (gray areas are seen dorsal to the optic disk) and followed by progressively increasing tapetal fundus hyperreflectivity that originates in the midperiphery and becomes generalized.

Retinal blood vessel attenuation occurs as in other forms of PRA.

ERGs of affected cats show responses of reduced amplitude and prolonged peak implicit times.

DIAGNOSIS

Breed incidence and age of onset of visual impairment and ophthalmoscopic changes
Electroretinography

DIFFERENTIAL DIAGNOSIS

Taurine deficiency retinopathy: cats of any breed fed a diet deficient in the amino acid taurine (dog food) may develop retinal degeneration. Ophthalmoscopically this has a characteristic appearance; it always begins in the area centralis and may or may not progress. The diagnosis here relies on history; check for any affected relatives, evidence of abnormal diet, or even test-mating.

TREATMENT

None. Avoid breeding from affected Abyssinian cats, their parents, and their progeny.

Gyrate Atrophy of the Retina and Choroid

Gyrate atrophy has been recorded in the cat. This is a metabolic disease caused by an inherited deficiency of the urea cycle enzyme ornithine transaminase. The result is hyperornithinemia with ornithenuria and retinal atrophy.

Noninherited Retinal Degenerations

These diseases are uncommon and result usually from dietary deficiencies or, rarely, drug toxicity.

Sudden Acquired Retinal Degeneration

This condition is characterized by acute onset and is discussed in detail earlier in this chapter.

Vitamin A Deficiency

This disorder is rare in the dog and cat. It may occur as a consequence of dietary deficiency of vitamin A or as a result of a fat malabsorption problem. Vitamin A is a precursor of the visual pigment rhodopsin.

CLINICAL FINDINGS

Nyctalopia (night blindness)
Rod and cone degeneration occurs, and there may also be other ocular effects, such as xerophthalmia (dry eye).

The tapetal fundus may change color early in vitamin A′ deficiency.

DIAGNOSIS

Evidence of dietary deficiency or malabsorption
Bilaterally symmetrical fundus changes and other ocular findings
Possible systemic signs

TREATMENT

If treated early with vitamin A supplementation, the changes are reversible. Damage to the optic nerve is irreversible.

Vitamin E Deficiency

Experimental vitamin E deficiency in dogs causes retinal degeneration very similar to central PRA (retinal pigment epithelial dystrophy) with degeneration of rod and cone photoreceptors and retinal pigment epithelium hypertrophy and migration.

Taurine Deficiency Retinopathy

Deficiency of the amino acid taurine will cause retinal degeneration in several species experimentally, but in practice it is usually seen only in the cat, which has a high retinal requirement for the sulfur-containing amino acid. In cats the disease is also known as feline central retinal degeneration (FCRD). It is seen in cats fed exclusively on dog food and also in those with a malabsorption problem. Ophthalmoscopic evidence of retinal degeneration develops only after the cat has been on a deficient diet for several months.

CLINICAL FINDINGS

Ophthalmoscopic changes develop before the animal shows noticeable visual impairment.

The initial fundus change is a bilaterally symmetrical, dark gray, oval area in the area centralis that quickly develops a hyperreflective center; this change may be very subtle and require reduced ophthalmoscope illumination in order to be visualized.

With progression, a gray linear, hyperreflective streak may be seen running transversely immediately superior to the optic disk from the nasal to the temporal tapetal fundus and joining the area centralis lesion. This corresponds to the cone density distribution of the feline retina (Figure 4-22,*B*).

If taurine deficiency continues, the hyperreflectivity spreads over a period of months and becomes generalized, retinal blood vessels become narrow and disappear, and optic atrophy is apparent with total blindness. If the deficiency is corrected, the lesions remain static but will not regress (Figure 4–22,*C*).

DIAGNOSIS

History of feeding cats on dog food or other strange diets; malabsorption from the alimentary tract

Characteristic bilaterally symmetrical ophthalmoscopic findings

Measurements of plasma taurine may reveal lowered levels of the amino acid (less than 20 nmol/ml). However, these tests are expensive.

DIFFERENTIAL DIAGNOSIS

Hereditary retinal dystrophies: breed incidence, age of onset, different ophthalmoscopic appearance (except in very advanced cases), and no evidence of dietary deficiency all serve to differentiate hereditary dystrophies from FCRD.

TREATMENT

Correct any dietary deficiency. If necessary, feed a taurine supplement. The prognosis is good if vision has not already been severely compromised.

Inflammatory Retinal Disease

The retina and choroid are so closely associated that inflammation of one tissue invariably results in accompanying inflammation of the neighboring tissue. Hence, the terms *chorioretinitis* and *retinochoroiditis* are both used, depending on which tissue is primarily affected.

ETIOLOGY

Although many of these cases are idiopathic, there are several known causes. In the dog, distemper, toxoplasmosis, leishmaniasis, the oculomycoses (blastomycosis, histoplasmosis, cryptococcosis, coccidioidomycosis, and geotrichosis), toxocariasis, prototheocosis, brucellosis, and Rocky Mountain spotted fever can be causes.

In the cat, toxoplasmosis, feline infectious peritonitis, feline leukemia virus, tuberculosis, and the oculomycoses

OPHTHALMOSCOPIC SIGNS OF ACTIVE CHORIORETINITIS

Fuzzy or blurred areas along the retinal blood vessels (gray or white foci with indistinct borders)

Dark discolored areas of the tapetal fundus with blurred margins and reduced reflectivity

Gray or white discoloration of the nontapetal fundus

Retinal edema and detachment
Preretinal exudates (gray or white areas)
Vitreous haze or flare

OPHTHALMOSCOPIC SIGNS OF INACTIVE CHORIORETINITIS

Areas of hyperreflectivity in the tapetal fundus that have distinct
borders separating them from normal fundus
Pigmentation within the area is often present in bizarre patterns.
Depigmented areas in the nontapetal fundus.
Retinal blood vessels crossing an area of healed chorioretinitis are
often narrowed and tortuous.

Vision is variably affected in these inflammatory diseases, depending on the extent of involvement of the retina and the degree of involvement of other ocular tissues, including the concurrent presence of optic neuritis or anterior uveitis, and involvement of the central nervous system.

DIAGNOSIS

Diagnosis of the etiology of chorioretinitis should not be attempted purely on the basis of the ophthalmoscopic appearance, but should include a general physical examination and laboratory aids, including serology, blood culture, and biopsy of involved tissues, including ocular paracentesis.

TREATMENT

Treat the primary cause if this can be determined.
Covering systemic antibiotics are useful. Diuretics are of value in the case of retinal edema or detachment.

Optic Nerve

Diseases of the optic nerve that cause chronic visual loss are very uncommon. Optic neuritis is characterized by an acute onset; recurrent episodes and the sequelae of optic atrophy may present as a chronic problem.

Neoplasms

Neoplasms involving the nerve (most commonly meningiomas) may cause gradually progressive visual impairment.

CLINICAL FINDINGS

The tumor may or may not be visible ophthalmoscopically, depending on its location, size, and rate of growth.
Papilledema may be present.

Invariably unilateral and tending to interrupt the direct pupillary light reflex, but not the consensual reflex in the affected eye

A visual field deficit may be detected (the animal bumps into objects on one side only).

If orbital, then the tumor usually causes some deviation of the globe and limitation of ocular movement.

Reticulosis of the central nervous system may invade the optic nerve and cause a granulomatous appearance of the optic disk or optic neuritis.

DIAGNOSIS

On the basis of the findings of ophthalmic examination

TREATMENT

Enucleation or exenteration is usually indicated if the tumor can be totally removed.

Papilledema

Papilledema in dogs may result from neoplasia of the optic nerve, orbital space-occupying lesions, intracranial tumors with raised CSF pressure, systemic toxicosis, systemic hypertension, ocular hypotension, pancreatitis, or acute glaucoma. Papilledema itself does not cause loss of vision, but it is often followed by optic atrophy with progressive visual impairment and even blindness.

OPHTHALMOSCOPIC APPEARANCE

In papilledema, the optic disk is swollen with blurred edges and engorged overlying blood vessels.

There are sometimes papillary and peripapillary hemorrhages, retinal edema, and detachment.

In optic atrophy, the optic disk is pale, small, and depressed but may subsequently become pigmented and appear darker than normal.

There may be peripapillary retinal atrophy (an irregular hyper-reflective area immediately superior to the disk).

TREATMENT

None. The primary cause should be pursued and addressed if possible.

Central Nervous System

Chronic visual loss due to CNS disease may be associated with neoplasia as described previously. Accompanying neurologic signs tend to be present, but this is not always the case.

Lysosomal storage diseases are recognized as an uncommon phenomenon in several species. They most frequently affect neuronal tissue. Because the retina and retinal pigment epithelium develop from the neuroectodermal embryonic optic cup, they can be involved in these disorders. Loss of vision in the lysosomal storage diseases is usually due to central involvement, although some ocular structures may show evidence of the disease, including corneal clouding and pale, scattered foci in the fundus due to accumulation of substances such as lipopigment in the retinal ganglion cells or cells of the retinal pigment epithelium. Apart from visual impairment, there are always other CNS signs and occasionally signs related to involvement of other organ systems. Lysosomal storage disorders usually have an hereditary nature, are often autosomal recessive, and are seen in young animals. Examples have been recorded in the dog (ceroid lipofuscinosis in the English Setter and Dalmatian; fucosidosis in the English Springer Spaniel) and the cat (gangliosidosis in the Siamese). The clinical hallmarks of these conditions include corneal opacities, visual impairment, and neurologic disorders.

5 | *Abnormal Appearance*

Beverley Cottrell and
Robert L. Peiffer, Jr.

When presented with a patient accompanied by the rather broad complaint of abnormal appearance to the adnexa and/or globe, the clinician should address the following questions:

1. What is the correct description of this abnormality in regard to tissue(s) of involvement and nature of the disorder?
2. What is the most likely cause?
3. How can the diagnosis be confirmed?
4. What is the appropriate treatment?

CONDITIONS INVOLVING THE ORBIT AND/OR GLOBE

Exophthalmos

Exophthalmos is an abnormal prominence of a normal-sized globe and is usually a unilateral condition. Although the term *proptosis* may be used synonymously, convention has led to the use of the latter term to describe globes displaced by trauma and orbital hemorrhage. The most challenging differential diagnosis is to distinguish if the globe is exophthalmic or megophthalmic (enlarged due to chronic glaucoma). In exophthalmos, the third eyelid is usually, but not invariably, prominent, the corneal diameter is the same as the follow eye (assuming that it is normal), secondary exposure keratitis may be present due to lagophthalmos, and IOP is normal to slightly elevated. With megophthalmos, the third eyelid is not prominent, the corneal diameter is greater than the fellow eye, secondary changes of chronic glaucoma are present, and IOP is usually elevated.

In animals presented with disparity of globe prominence, apparently exophthalmic globes must be distinguished from normal globes with enophthalmic fellow eyes. With enophthalmos, the third eyelid is prominent; looking from above, the corneal apex may not be visible. Corneal diameter may be normal or reduced if the globe is microphthalmic or phthisical. Enophthalmos may be accompanied by other signs, as in Horner's syndrome.

Bilateral cases of exophthalmos are uncommon: brachycephalics (Pug, Lhasa Apso) have a shallow orbit and a relatively large eye. This condition predisposes to traumatic proptosis and chronic keratitis but is normal for the breed.

Exophthalmos is caused by space-occupying lesions of the orbit or periorbital tissues, most commonly inflammation or neoplasia. Orbital inflammation may be diffuse (cellulitis) or localized as an abscess. Clinical signs usually include a history of acute onset, pain on retropulsion of globe and on opening the mouth, lethargy, depression, and inappetence. Pyrexia, neutrophilia, chemosis, prominence of the third eyelid, impaired eye movements, and deviation of the globe are variable observations. Occasionally anterior drainage through the conjunctiva will occur. Etiology includes foreign bodies (including grass awns and fragments of stick or bone that may enter behind the last molar tooth), dental disease (tooth root abscess), zygomatic adenitis, or hematogenous or local spread of an infectious agent. Diagnosis is made based upon history and clinical examination; hematology, radiography, and aspiration biopsy may provide insight into individual nonresponsive cases. Treatment involves systemic antibiotics for ten days; one should see a rapid and permanent improvement. Surgical drainage via the oral cavity is indicated in chronic or recurrent cases, and surgical exploration is indicated in tracts draining through the conjunctiva.

Orbital neoplasia may be primary or secondary, the latter due to extension from the nasal chambers and/or paranasal sinuses or metastases from distant sites. Clinical signs include a slow onset with absence of pain, progressive globe deviation, and third eyelid prominence (depending upon position of the tumor) and may include bony swelling and facial deformities (Figure 5–1). Exposure keratitis may be present if lagophthalmos is present. Diagnosis is based on history, clinical examination, radiography, and biopsy by aspiration or exploratory surgery. Treatment may be frustrating, as the majority of primary tumors are aggressively invasive malignancies that are diagnosed at an advanced stage. In general, these cases are best managed by an ophthalmologist and/or oncologist.

Other causes of exophthalmos that should be included in a differential diagnosis include posterior scleritis; orbital cysts, congenital or acquired; eosinophilic myositis (swelling of masticatory muscles forces orbital fat forwards); arteriovenous shunt; emphysema (from fractures of the paranasal sinuses); hemorrhage (trauma, blood dyscrasias); and edema (associated with estrus, migrating *Dirofilaria*, hypoproteinemia, or systemic hypertension). Standard methods are used to define and treat these uncommon

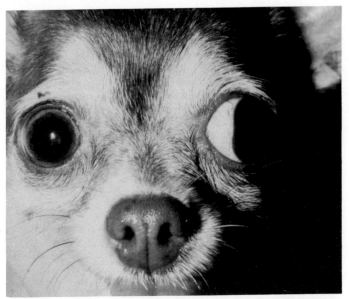

FIGURE 5-1. Exophthalmos, left eye, in a 10-year-old Chihuahua with an orbital neoplasm. The globe is deviated temporally (exotropia), and there was resistance to retropulsion.

causes of exophthalmos; challenging diagnostic cases should be referred to a specialist for consideration of such techniques as ultrasound, orbital imaging, and exploratory orbitotomy.

Traumatic Proptosis

Blunt or penetrating trauma to the head can result in forceful anterior displacement of the globe. Prognosis is related to breed, duration, and associated complications. In the brachycephalic breeds of dogs, the problem can occur with a minimum of trauma. In other dogs and cats, proptosis is more likely to be accompanied by severe head trauma and orbital hemorrhage. Management of the proptosis should be undertaken with a "whole animal" perspective.

Rapid replacement of the globe is the most important aspect of management. Several pathologic processes occur as a result of proptosis; the exposed tissue will quickly desiccate, and protection with a moist gauze or cloth prior to correction can be instructed over the telephone and initiated by the client on the way to the surgery. Constriction of the eyelids behind the globe not only makes replacement difficult but also may cause vascular strangulation with resultant ischemic necrosis of ocular tissues. Stretching of the optic nerve and extraocular muscles may result in rupture of these tissues, and damage to orbital vasculature results in orbital hemorrhage that will make replacement challenging. The globe itself may have been ruptured by the traumatic event.

If the globe is ruptured or the optic nerve and/or ocular vasculature is severed, enucleation is indicated. Otherwise, replacement should be attempted. Pupillary light reflexes are not always a reliable prognosticator; optic nerve damage may be transient or a traumatic uveitis may cause miosis. A guarded visual prognosis should always be given in complicated or prolonged cases. In uncomplicated cases in brachycephalics, with topical anesthesia, manual retraction of the eyelids, and posterior pressure on the globe through moistened gauze, replacement is usually readily accomplished. Otherwise, under short-acting general anesthesia, a muscle hook is used to "tire rim" the eyelids from behind the globe. If orbital hemorrhage is severe and/or replacement difficult, a lateral canthotomy should be utilized. A temporary tarsorrhaphy should be performed and left in place for at least one week. Apply topical antibiotic and atropine ointments prior to closing the tarsorrhaphy. Postoperative systemic corticosteroids (for optic neuritis) and antibiotics are indicated.

Sequelae include optic atrophy (common); strabismus due to rupture of the extraocular muscles (usually the medial rectus is involved, with resultant exotropia); or keratoconjunctivitis sicca (uncommon). Strabismus usually improves over time, although surgical repair may be attempted by an ophthalmologist.

Enophthalmos

Enophthalmos is abnormal retraction or "sinking" of a normal-sized globe into the orbit. Clinically, the distinction between enophthalmos and microphthalmia or phthisis bulbi is important. With enophthalmos, the corneal diameter is the same as the fellow eye (assuming that is normal); the third eyelid is usually prominent, passively prolapsing as resistance from the globe is withdrawn; and the globe is normal in all other respects (although Horner's syndrome is accompanied by miosis). There is usually no deviation or nystagmus. With microphthalmos, history will indicate a congenital problem. The corneal diameter is less than the fellow eye, the third eyelid is usually prominent, and the globe may show other abnormalities such as cataract, poor limbal differentiation, rotatory nystagmus, or persistent pupillary membranes. Phthisis bulbi will be accompanied by a history of an acquired condition secondary to trauma or inflammation. IOP will be low and the cornea opaque.

Pseudoenophthalmos may result from periorbital swelling and blepharoconjunctival edema: this distinction can be made by examination of the adnexa.

Physiologic enophthalmos is congenital and associated with dolichocephalics, including Collies and Dobermans. In addition to deep orbits, these dogs often have a relatively small eye, which accentuates the enophthalmos. Secondary changes may be present, including mucus accumulation at the medial canthus, epiphora, chronic conjunctivitis, and occasionally entropion.

Enophthalmos may be active or passive. The most common causes of active enophthalmos, which is due to contraction of the retractor oculi muscle, are pain and tetanus. The retractor oculi muscle in the dog pulls the eye into the orbit when pain is present; this muscle is not as active in the cat. Check for distichiasis and ectopic cilia, foreign bodies, and intraocular disease. General anesthesia may be necessary to examine the eye adequately. Treatment depends upon identifying and treating the primary cause; the enophthalmos should then resolve. Enophthalmos in tetanus is bilateral and is caused by spasm of the retractor oculi muscles. Diagnose and treat according to standard methods.

The most common causes of passive enophthalmos are loss of retrobulbar fat secondary to inflammation or chronic wasting and Horner's syndrome. Loss of retrobulbar fat causes a mechanical sinking of the globe into the orbit. This fact may be lost as a result of systemic disease (especially vomiting, diarrhea, and subsequent dehydration and/or generalized weight loss) as well as orbital or periorbital postinflammatory atrophy. It may also be lost as a result of senility; progressive bilateral enophthalmos is not an uncommon feature of aging in dogs. History and clinical examination should make the diagnosis obvious. Treatment depends upon identifying the primary cause.

The signs of Horner's syndrome are caused by interruption to the sympathetic nervous supply to the eye and include enophthalmos, miosis, protrusion of the third eyelid, ptosis (drooping of the upper lid), and conjunctival vasodilation. The condition is by far most commonly unilateral but may be bilateral. Besides the relative miosis, ocular examination is unremarkable. Comparison with the fellow eye is helpful in making this observation.

Other causes of enophthalmos include traumatic periorbital tears (traumatic tears in the ventral periorbita allow the globe to move ventrally in the pterygopalatine fossa; refer these cases to a specialist for repair); globe perforation (digital palpation should reveal a hypotensive globe; the laceration should be repaired as an emergency); and periorbital muscle atrophy, most commonly following eosinophilic myositis. The acute stages may be characterized by exophthalmos; muscle biopsy should confirm the diagnosis.

Megophthalmos

Megophthalmos is an increase in the size of the globe secondary to chronic glaucoma, the cornea and sclera stretching in response to elevated IOP, and is associated with loss of vision. Young animals have less scleral rigidity and are prone to the condition. Synonyms include *hydrophthalmos, buphthalmos, megalophthalmos,* and *megaloglobus*. In arriving at this diagnosis, the clinician should determine whether the globe is megophthalmic or exophthalmic, and if the apparently affected globe is truly megophthalmic or if the apparently normal globe is microphthalmic or enophthalmic. Megophthalmos is always accompanied by secondary changes, which may include episcleral injection, corneal edema, Descemet's fractures, scleral ectasia (thinning) giving a bluish appearance, a fixed dilated pupil, and lens subluxation/luxation, and by glaucomatous retinal and optic atrophy. IOP may or may not be elevated, and exposure keratitis may or may not be present. Specific signs depend on the pathogenesis, severity, and duration of the glaucoma.

Treatment is indicated if the eye is painful or unsightly, or if an intraocular tumor is suspected. Many animals not obviously uncomfortable benefit from therapy with notable improvement in personality. Systemic and topical ocular hypotensive medication is generally ineffective. Although topical ointments may provide relief from exposure, definitive reduction of IOP is best accomplished by surgical means; enucleation, cyclocryosurgery, evisceration with insertion of an intraocular prosthesis, or intraocular injection of gentamicin are all reasonable alternatives. If an intraocular tumor is suspected, enucleation is indicated.

Microphthalmos and Nanophthalmos

Microphthalmos is a congenitally abnormally small eye with multiple anomalies that generally render the globe sightless; *nanophthalmos* is a small but otherwise structurally and functionally normal globe. The condition is hereditary in some breeds (Doberman, Australian Shepherd, West Highland White Terrier, Old English Sheepdog) and is seen in the Miniature Schnauzer associated with congenital cataracts. True *anophthalmos*, or complete absence of the eye, is extremely rare.

With unilateral cases, differential diagnosis warrants the following considerations: Is the eye truly microphthalmic or is its fellow megophthalmic? Is the eye microphthalmic or enophthalmic?

Microphthalmos is frequently accompanied by cataract, persistent pupillary membranes, lens coloboma, poor limbal differentiation, and rotatory nystagmus. Distinction from phthisis bulbi may be difficult but can usually be surmised based on history (age of onset, previous trauma, or inflammation). Bilateral cases of nanophthalmos may be related to breed standards (Collie, Shetland Sheepdog, Bullmastiff). Normal-sized globes may be apparently nanophthalmic because of periorbital fat (Shar Pei, Chow Chow).

No treatment is available. Because of the potential for genetic transmission, dogs affected with microphthalmos should not be bred.

Phthisis bulbi

Phthisis bulbi is an acquired degenerate eye and represents a nonspecific end stage of a severe intraocular disease, such as glaucoma, trauma, or inflammation; injury to the ciliary body results in cessation of aqueous production. The globe then shrinks and atrophies. Distinction from microphthalmos can generally be made based on history and measurement of IOP, which is more likely to be low in phthisical globes.

Visual prognosis is grave once shrinkage has begun. With early phthisis, evisceration and insertion of an intraocular prosthesis will provide the best cosmetic result. These animals are predisposed to chronic conjunctivitis as ocular secretions pool in the enlarged inferior fornix; regular irrigation and topical antibiotics and/or corticosteroids as needed provide relief. Enucleation is recommended if the conjunctivitis is severe and intractable. In cats, phthisical globes should be enucleated because of the propensity for primary ocular sarcomas to develop.

Neurological Syndromes

Neurological disorders may underlie many ocular conditions, including abnormalities in pupil size, with resultant abnormal appearance.

Horner's Syndrome

The signs of Horner's syndrome, discussed previously in this chapter in relation to enophthalmos, are caused by an interruption to the sympathetic nervous supply of the eye (Figure 5-2). The sympathetic pathway involves both central and peripheral components, and disruption of the pathway at any level may result in Horner's syndrome. Depending upon the level of the lesion, Horner's may be classified as first, second, or third order.

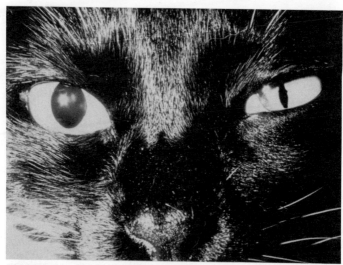

FIGURE 5–2. Horner's syndrome of the left eye in a domestic shorthair; ptosis, relative miosis, prolapse of the third eyelid, and apparent enophthalmos are observed. Note the absence of signs of inflammation or pain.

First-order Horner's is uncommon and involves first-order neurons—a central lesion prior to synapse in the thoracic spinal cord. The condition may be cerebral, brain stem, or thoracic and is almost always accompanied by other neurological signs. Second-order Horner's involves second-order preganglionic neurons. The lesion may be cranial thoracic, in the neck, or a soft tissue lesion close to the carotid artery or middle ear; choke chain trauma is a common cause. Usually no other ophthalmic or neurologic signs are present. Third-order Horner's involves third-order postganglionic neurons. The usual cause is orbital disease, and the condition is usually accompanied by other ophthalmic or neurological signs, including nystagmus or abnormal tonic eye reflexes. Establishing which order is present is important so that the level of the lesion can be pinpointed. Upon clinical diagnosis of Horner's syndrome based upon the classical signs (ptosis, relative miosis, enophthalmos, and protrusion of the third eyelid), a detailed neurological examination is indicated. Thoracic, head, and neck radiographs should be undertaken. In cases of first-order Horner's, CSF examination may be helpful.

Topical pharmacologic agents will assist in determination of order (Figure 5–3). Topical 1.5% cocaine will dilate a normal pupil but not a Horner's pupil; 1% hydroxyamphetamine will dilate a first- or second-order Horner's pupil but not a third order; 10%

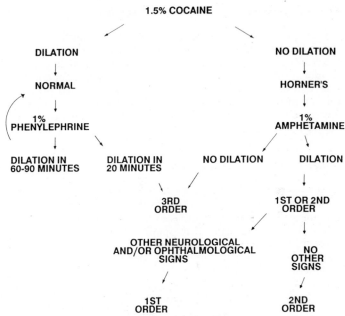

FIGURE 5-3. Horner's syndrome—which order?

phenylephrine hydrochloride will dilate a third-order pupil in 20 minutes, but a normal pupil will dilate only after 60 to 90 minutes.

Remember that when considering a clinical diagnosis of Horner's syndrome, bilateral enophthalmos and third eyelid prominence may be due to dehydration, especially in cats; such cases show no miosis. Miosis in Horner's syndrome is relative; the anisocoria, as well as the ptosis, may be subtle. The typical Horner's pupil will fail to dilate in dim light conditions. Miosis alone may be caused by orbital or CNS trauma or by anterior uveitis.

Symptomatic treatment of Horner's syndrome involves topical 0.1% epinephrine drops or 0.12% phenylephrine drops to effect (start off twice daily). These drops are somewhat irritating, and treatment is recommended only if eyelid protrusion impairs visual function. If the primary cause is identified and amenable to treatment, of course, such treatment should be considered.

Prognosis is dependent on cause; in general, the more peripheral a traumatic lesion (second and third order), the more likely spontaneous resolution will occur, although it may require several months.

Feline Dysautonomia (Key-Gaskell Syndrome)

Described in the United Kingdom and other countries, the condition is rare in the United States, and incidence is decreasing. Signs are referable to parasympathetic loss and include pupillary dilation, protrusion of the third eyelid, systemic signs of constipation, and regurgitation. The etiology is unknown, and prognosis for complete recovery is very poor. Treatment includes oral pilocarpine drops twice daily, stool softeners for constipation, and tender loving care and constant nursing.

Other Disorders of Anisocoria

Anisocoria is a difference in the size of the pupils. Deciding which pupil is abnormal is critical: is the correct diagnosis unilateral miosis or unilateral mydriasis? If the pupil is miotic, it will fail to dilate in dim light. If the pupil is mydriatic, it will fail to constrict in bright light. Consideration of the cause of anisocoria includes ocular and neurological conditions; ocular conditions include iritis (miosis); traumatic rupture of the sphincter muscle (mydriasis); glaucoma (mydriasis); iris atrophy (mydriasis); and retinal or optic disk lesions (mydriasis). Neurological disease involving the afferent arc, such as optic neuritis or a compressive chiasmatic lesion, will result in mydriasis. Lesions of the oculomotor nucleus and nerve may be irritative (miosis) or destructive (mydriasis). Confirm the diagnosis by exclusion, and treat according to etiology.

Strabismus

Strabismus is an abnormal alignment of the eye(s) in which the visual axes are not parallel. Strabismus may be classified as convergent (esotropic) or divergent (exotropic); unilateral (one eye used for fixation) or bilateral (eyes used alternately or equally); and incomitant (deviation varies according to position of gaze) or concomitant (deviation is similar in all directions).

Causes include heredity (esotropia in Siamese cats, an autosomal recessive trait, or exotropia in brachycephalic breeds); post-traumatic proptosis due to rupture of the extraocular muscles, most commonly the medial rectus with a unilateral divergent concomitant strabimus; extraocular muscle paresis (incomitant); and severe visual deficit (concomitant), either congenital or acquired. Clinical examination and history should confirm the diagnosis.

Corrective surgery by a specialist is possible although usually not required for adequate visual function.

EYELIDS

Ophthalmia Neonatorum

This condition is due to purulent keratoconjunctivitis in the neonate occurring before the lids open and is manifested by unilateral or bilateral swelling with or without purulent discharge at the medial canthus. The most likely causes include staphylococcal infection in the dog (which may be acquired in utero) and viral infections in the cat, especially with herpes and/or calicivirus. An unlikely differential diagnosis should include congenital glaucoma.

Diagnosis is confirmed by gentle separation of the lids either manually or surgically, depending upon age. Treatment should be immediate and aggressive and include irrigation with sterile saline and frequent topical antibiotics and lubricants. Systemic antibiotics are indicated with globe perforation or risk of perforation. Regular cleaning is important to prevent readherence of lids. Prognosis is guarded as secondary changes, including corneal scarring, ulceration, perforation, and symblepharon, are common.

Dermoids

Hamartomatous proliferations may result in focal thickening and misdirection of eyelid hair (Figure 5-4). Although eyelid dermoids may be excised if trichiasis results, most are well tolerated and require no therapy.

Ectropion

Ectropion is an eversion of the eyelid (usually lower), exposing palpebral and bulbar conjunctiva. The condition is hereditary in certain breeds, including the American Cocker Spaniel, Basset Hound, and Bloodhound. Animals with weak lateral control support structures (the St. Bernard and other giant breeds are predisposed) have diamond-shaped palpebral fissures with medial and lateral entropion and central ectropion. Ectropion may occur intermittently in any breed following exercise. The condition may be associated with senile atrophy of the orbicularis muscle (frequently accompanied by senile entropion of the upper lid) or secondary to trauma (including overcorrection of entropion).

Treatment is seldom indicated for simple ectropion; chronic conjunctivitis is usually manageable with daily lavage with sterile saline and topical antibiotics and corticosteroids as required. In giant breeds with combined entropion-ectropion, reconstruction of the lateral canthal ligament is indicated. The *V-Y* procedure is

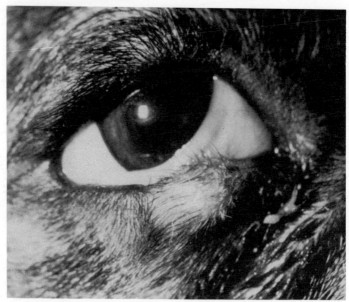

FIGURE 5-4. Eyelid dermoid, lower right lid, in a Boxer pup.

effective in the management of cicatrical entropion, and various lid-shortening and tightening procedures can be used to repair primary ectropion if required.

Agenesis (Lid Coloboma, Eyelid Dysgenesis)

This is an uncommon condition seen mainly as a bilateral congenital anomaly in cats and involves absence of part or all of the eyelid margin; the superior temporal lid is most commonly involved (Figure 5-5). The condition is also seen in the Staffordshire Bull Terrier in association with corneal and conjunctival dermoids. Exposure and irritation (trichiasis) invariably result in keratoconjunctivitis.

Corrective surgery is possible; the "bucket-handle" technique provides consistently good results (see Figure 5-7). This extensive blepharoplasty is best handled by a specialist.

Blepharitis

Inflammation of the skin of the eyelid is usually a disease of young animals and infectious (bacterial *Staphylococcus;* fungal *Trichophyton* or *Microsporum;* parasitic *Demodex* or *Sar-*

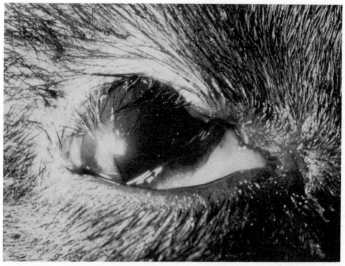

FIGURE 5-5. Eyelid agenesis in a young domestic shorthair. The superior temporal margin is absent, with resultant trichiasis.

coptes) in cause. The condition is usually associated with some degree of keratoconjunctivitis. Other causes include generalized dermatologic disease, such as seborrhea, atopy, and other immune-mediated processes, trauma (including self-trauma), and neoplasia of the lids.

Diagnosis is made by clinical evidence of eyelid inflammation and etiology determined by standard methods, including skin scraping and biopsy.

Symptomatic therapy involves regular irrigation and hot packs to keep the lids free of exudate and topical and/or systemic medication directed toward the etiology.

Chalazion and Hordeolum

Inflammation of the meibomian glands may be acute (meibomianitis, internal hordeolum) or chronic (chalazion) and appear as localized areas of inflammation most obvious on the palpebral surface of the eyelid. An external hordeolum or stye is an infection of a lash follicle and associated sebaceous glands and presents as an area of localized inflammation at the lid margin.

Acute meibomianitis manifests as conjunctivitis with linear yellow-white swellings perpendicular to the lid margin seen on eversion of the lid. The swelling is due to inspissated meibomian secretions and/or purulent exudate. The condition is painful and may coexist with other inflammatory conditions such as KCS or blepharitis. A chalazion presents as a small, round swelling visible under the skin and is more obvious from the conjunctival surface when the lid is everted as a localized, yellowish, elevated lesion. The condition is painless, and the overlying palpebral conjunctiva may be hyperemic. The lesion is hard on palpation and will not markedly increase in size over time. Pathogenesis likely involves infection with resultant obstruction of the meibomian ducts. As the secretory material accumulates, it elicits a granulomatous inflammatory response.

An external hordeolum is an acute infection (usually staphylococcal) resulting in localized swelling of the lid margin. The condition is seen in young animals, may be associated with blepharitis, and is painful (thus accompanied by blepharospasm and lacrimation). Meibomianitis and external hordeolum are best managed by hot compresses and topical antibiotics. Chalazion and nonresponsive cases should be incised and curetted. A chalazion clamp facilitates either procedure; histopathology of curretted tissue is recommended.

Neoplasia

Eyelid tumors have species-specific characteristics; in the dog, most are of meibomian sebaceous gland origin (adenoma); papillomas and melanomas are also common, and almost all are benign. In the cat, squamous cell carcinoma and sarcomas, both aggressive malignancies, are the rule. Eyelid tumors may cause secondary irritation and may present with keratoconjunctivitis and/or ocular discharge.

Clinical appearance will provide clues to the type of tumor. Adenomas usually involve the meibomian gland and thus the eyelid margin and tarsoconjunctiva; these may or may not be pigmented. Melanomas have variable appearance but frequently involve the lid margin only. Papillomas are seen in young dogs (with or without oral papillomatosis) and are unpigmented with an irregular surface; they may or may not arise from the lid margin. Squamous cell carcinomas present as ulcerative, invasive, and destructive lesions.

Treatment is indicated for irritative marginal lesions and tumors with a documented increase in size over time. Full-thickness excision with repair in two layers (tarsoconjunctiva and skin) ensuring good lid margin apposition and 2- 3-mm surgical margins is recommended; up to one-third of the lid can be removed and primarily closed in dogs (depending on breed); the "tight" lids of the cat are somewhat less forgiving (Figure 5–6). Several blepharoplastic techniques are available for more extensive tumors; we

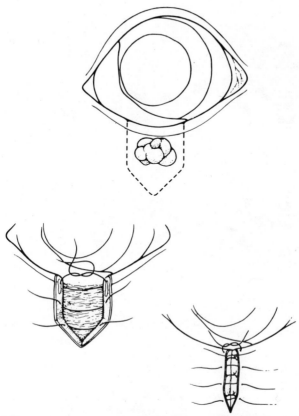

FIGURE 5–6. Pentagonal wedge resection for eyelid neoplasms. A scalpel is used to delineate the extent of the resection and incise the skin; scissors are used to complete the excision. Two-layer closure with a 4-0 or 5-0 absorbable suture with buried knots placed through the tarsoconjunctiva and similar-sized nonabsorbable suture placed through the skin is utilized. Accurate apposition of the eyelid margin is of paramount concern. The pentagonal excision distributes suture tension more evenly than a three-sided excision. From Peiffer RL Jr et al: Surgery of the canine and feline orbit, adnexa, and globe. Part III: Other structural abnormalities in neoplasia of the eyelids. *Companion Animal Practice* 1:20–36, September 1987.

have found the bucket-handle technique to be a versatile and effective technique (Figure 5–7).

Cryosurgery is effective alternative to surgical excision; small tumors may be treated with local anesthesia on an outpatient basis.

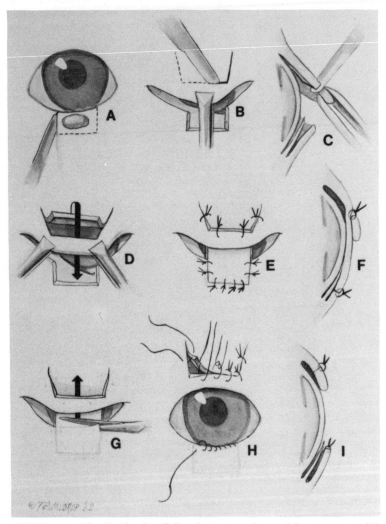

FIGURE 5–7. The "bucket-handle" technique can be useful to repair eyelid agenesis in cats or large lid defects following excision of tumors. A two-stage procedure, its advantage lies in the fact that both conjunctival and epidermal tissues are grafted; it works equally well for upper-to-lower and lower-to-upper lid grafting. *A,* Large, full-thickness lower eyelid defect is excised "en bloc."

B, A full-thickness advancement flap is fashioned from the upper lid above a 4-mm bridge of lid margin. The flap is constructed slightly wider than the defect and is broader at its base than at the free margin. The bridge must be wide enough to maintain its vitality and is handled minimally and atraumatically.

Larger masses likewise respond remarkably well. Healing is by secondary intention but cosmetic and functional results are usually good (Figure 5-8). Follow general principles for cryosurgery of neoplasms; care should be taken to protect the globe.

Supplementary oncotherapy may be considered in extensive cases, notably radiation therapy for squamous cell carcinomas.

Traumatic Eyelid Injuries

Traumatic injuries are generally mechanical in nature and can be divided clinically into those that involve only the eyelid and those that involve the full thickness of the eyelid. Principles established for the management of traumatic lesions elsewhere in the body are applicable to the eyelids and include copious irrigation, minimal debridement, and plastic repair to restore anatomic and functional integrity. In any type of traumatic injury to the lids, the globe should be carefully examined to determine the presence or absence of concurrent ocular involvement.

Pruritic dermatologic conditions often result in self-trauma to the area; this excoriation is best managed by treatment of the initiating factors. Abrasions of the eyelids are uncommon but heal readily. Most commonly, traumatic injuries are lacerations related to skirmishes with other dogs and cats.

C, Tarsoconjunctiva and skin-orbicularis layers are identified in both the recipient and donor tissues; blunt subcutaneous dissection may be performed to mobilize the upper lid flap, and, if necessary, a lower lid advancement flap may be prepared.

D, The flap is pulled beneath the bridge and the tarsoconjunctiva sutured to the identical layer of the defect. Size 4-0 (1.5 metric) absorbable suture is used, and the knots tied on the tarsal surface.

E,F, In a similar fashion the skin-orbicularis layers are united with 4-0 (1.5 metric) nonabsorbable suture. The raw edges of bridge and flap in the upper lid may be sutured to minimize tension, and a temporary tarsorrhaphy may be performed along the intact lid margin. The exposed surfaces are kept moist with topical antibiotic ointments or dressings.

G, After 3 to 4 weeks, the sutures are removed and the new lid margin is formed by incision under general anesthesia. The advancement flap is freed, the margins of the bridge are minimally debrided, and the upper lid is restored with a routine two layer closure. Conjunctiva and skin layers of the new lower eyelid margin are joined with continuous suture; size 6-0 (0.7 metric) absorbable sutures are preferred. Skin sutures placed at this time are removed in 7 to 10 days. Residual marginal trichiasis is managed by using an entropion repair to redirect the hairs. From Peiffer RL Jr et al: Surgery of the canine and feline orbit, adnexa, and globe. Part III: Other structural abnormalities and neoplasia of the eyelids. *Companion Animal Practice* 1:20–36, September 1987.

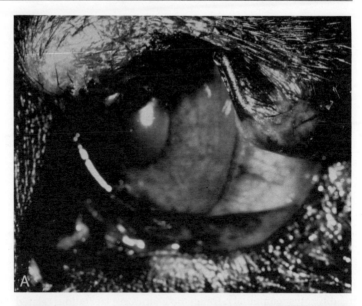

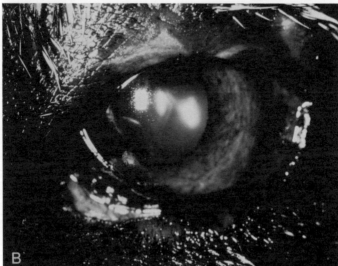

FIGURE 5-8. Large meibomian adenomas treated by cryosurgery in an elderly, overweight Doberman, preoperatively (*A*) and four months following surgery (*B*). Loss of eyelid hair and skin depigmentation are anticipated complications.

The eyelids are highly vascular structures and demonstrate remarkable capacities for healing and resistance to infection. Eyelids that are almost completely avulsed can be successfully repaired simply by suturing them back into the proper position as soon after injury as possible. Three principles should guide correction of eyelid lacerations.

1. Direct closure and healing by primary intention will provide the most consistent satisfactory results. To delay operation on a traumatized eyelid will result in surgery on distorted and possibly infected tissues, necessitating more extensive debridement.

2. Of primary concern is restoration of the eyelid margin and the palpebral fissure.

3. The tarsus is the layer of maximal suture-holding strength; two-layer closure is the closure technique of choice.

The lacrimal puncta and canaliculi should be identified and preserved if possible; epiphora may be a postoperative complication if the punctum (especially the lower) is occluded in healing. Possible sequelae of deep lacerations to the face around the lids include ectropion or entropion as these wounds contract; the lid malformation is managed surgically as a secondary procedure following complete healing of the initial wound.

CONJUNCTIVA

Hemorrhage

Subconjunctival hemorrhage may be traumatic, in which case it tends to be diffuse and extensive, or occur secondary to a systemic clotting deficiency, in which cases discrete petechiae or ecchymoses are observed. Occasionally conjunctival hemorrhage can be associated with infectious agents, notably *Rickettsia*.

In cases of traumatic subconjunctival hemorrhage, clinical examination should differentiate between uncomplicated subconjunctival hemorrhage and subconjunctival hemorrhage occurring with extensive orbital hemorrhage. In the latter case, exophthalmos and resistance to retropulsion of the globe will be noted. Rupture of the globe posterior to the limbus should also be considered; it can be detected by the presence of an extremely low intraocular pressure.

Uncomplicated hemorrhage resolves spontaneously without therapy; if orbital hemorrhage is present, protection of the cornea with lubricants and/or temporary tarsorrhaphy should be considered during the resorption process, which may take up to several weeks.

Hyperemia

Conjunctival hyperemia is one of the main reasons why animals are presented with a "red eye"; the main clinical distinction is separating conjunctival hyperemia, almost invariably associated with inflammation, from hyperemia of the deeper episcleral vessels, which is generally associated with more serious, deeper disease processes (conjunctival hyperemia and episcleral injection can occur simultaneously).

Conjunctival hyperemia is more intense at the fornix, characterized by dilated arborescent blood vessels that move when the conjunctiva is moved, and are bright red in appearance. Topical epinephrine will cause prompt and dramatic blanching of conjunctival vessels. Episcleral or ciliary injection is more intense at the limbus; the vessels tend to be straight, remain stationary when the conjunctiva is moved, are deeper red in color, and do not as readily blanch with topical epinephrine. Episcleral injection is frequently associated with glaucoma, uveitis, or intraocular neoplasia.

True conjunctival hyperemia can be passive, occurring secondarily to impaired local or systemic circulation, such as is seen in venous congestion due to heart failure or increased blood viscosity due to dehydration or multiple myeloma. In systemic toxemias, the conjunctiva frequently appears brick red as an indicator of panvascular affects. Active hyperemia is associated with an inflammatory response; etiologies might include irritative conditions such as distichiasis or foreign bodies, keratoconjunctivitis sicca, or infectious conjunctivitis. In general, conjunctivitis is characterized by exudation, and is discussed in detail in Chapter 7 on ocular discharge.

Membranous Conjunctivitis

An uncommon disease presumed to be an immunorelated process is seen in Doberman Pinschers and Golden Retrievers. The ocular lesions appear as a bilateral yellow-green membrane lining any or all of the conjunctival surfaces; stripping the ulcer away leaves a roughened and ulcerated epithelial surface. Exfoliative cytology reveals inflammatory cells with a prominent eosinophilic component; the membrane itself is composed of epithelial cells and a proteinaceous exudate. Variable associated systemic signs include proteinuria and ulcerative lesions of the skin and other mucus membranes, notably the oral cavity. This enigmatic condition can be controlled in most cases with topical corticosteroids as well as systemic corticosteroids and/or azothioprine.

Tumors

Conjunctival tumors are uncommon and may be classified as inflammatory or neoplastic. The same group of immune-mediated granulomatous inflammatory conditions that affect the cornea and nictitating membrane can involve the episcleral and manifest as subconjunctival masses. Primary conjunctival tumors are uncommon in the dog and cat and include papilloma, hemangioma, and melanoma. The most common secondary tumor is lymphosarcoma. Treatment is by biopsy, excisional if possible, and definitive diagnosis is dependent upon histopathologic examination.

Cystic lesions of the conjunctiva may be seen in young dogs, most likely associated with congenitally ectopic glandular tissue or occluded ducts. Frequently aspiration of the clear fluid is curative; if not, excision is easily performed.

Symblepharon

Symblepharon is adhesion of the conjunctiva to itself, with obliteration of the fornices, or to the corneal surface. Frequently, the nasolacrimal puncta will be destroyed by the scarring, and the adhesions may cause the third eyelid to remain in a prolapsed position. The condition is by far most commonly encountered in the cat, in which it is likely to occur secondary to ophthalmia neonatorium or upper respiratory-associated infectious keratoconjunctivitis. The condition is generally painless, but epiphora and a mild, persistent conjunctivitis may be present. Upon careful examination and probing, the fornices are usually obliterated or reduced in depth; corneal involvement requires differentiation from a vascular keratitis. Corneal symblepharon can be elevated from the surface with fine-toothed forceps and topical anesthesia. Mild cases need not be treated; if vision is significantly impaired, plastic surgical reconstruction can be attempted by a specialist. However, because of the tendency for adhesions to reform, prognosis is not always favorable.

Pigmentation

Conjunctival pigmentation is almost always associated with melanin deposition within the conjunctival epithelium and/or proliferation of melanocytes in the subepithelial stroma. Slight pigmentation is a normal finding; exaggeration is almost always associated with chronic irritation, including exposure, and is frequently seen within the palpebral fissure of brachycephalic breeds. Malignant melanomas of the conjunctiva are exceedingly rare; if a pigmented area is observed to be elevated in a nodular fashion and/or to increase in size over time, excisional biopsy is indicated. Limbal melanocytomas in the dog and cat as well as anterior uveal melanomas in the dog frequently present as subconjunctival nodular pigmented masses; they are discussed in detail later in this chapter.

THIRD EYELID

Several conditions result in abnormal prominence and/or appearance of the third eyelid.

Prolapse of the Gland of the Third Eyelid

The gland of the third eyelid surrounds the base of the T-shaped support cartilage, presumably fixed by soft tissue to the deep corrective tissue. In this condition, commonly referred to as *cherry eye*, the base of the gland everts (presumably due to hypoplasia of fascial adhesions) to protrude as a smooth pink mass above the leading edge of the membrane. Secondary conjunctivitis may occur, and eversion of the cartilage occasionally accompanies it. The condition is probably inherited and occurs in young dogs, with the Beagle, American Cocker Spaniel, St. Bernard, Weimaraner, and English Bulldog predisposed. The condition occurs rarely in the cat. The condition may be unilateral or bilateral and not always concurrently so.

Diagnosis involves differentiation from neoplasia of the gland (seen in older dogs) and congenital cysts; age will usually allow distinction of the former, and transillumination and/or aspiration usually distinguishes of the latter.

The classical method of treatment—excision of the prolapsed gland—is not recommended, as this gland produces about one-third of the aqueous tears, and removal predisposes the animal to KCS later in life. Surgical replacement involves suturing the gland back in position and is a reliable, effective procedure (Figure 5–9).

Eversion of Cartilage

In this condition, the free edge of the membrane rolls outwards from the globe to scroll upon itself; the condition is usually associated with a mild exposure conjunctivitis. A predisposition for the giant canine breeds exists; cartilage eversion occurs usually in young dogs (less than one year) but is not usually congenital. The condition may be unilateral or bilateral.

Iatrogenic eversion may be caused by damage to cartilage through careless suturing of third eyelid flaps; careful suture placement and control of tension will avoid this problem.

Treatment involves surgical removal of the buckled cartilage under general anesthesia (Figure 5–10).

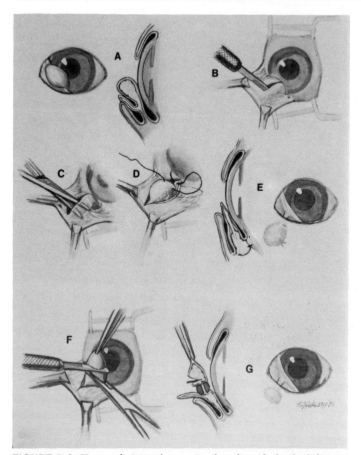

FIGURE 5-9. Two techniques for repair of prolapsed gland of the nictitating membrane: suture adenopexy and partial incision. *A,* Prolapse of the gland of the nictitating membrane up and over the free edge. *B,* Incision through the bulbar mucosa of the membrane. *C,* Dissection of the mucosa overlying the gland. *D,* The globe is rotated dorsally and a 4-0 absorbable mattress suture is placed on the inferior nasalbulbar fascia and the prolapsed base of the gland. *E,* The gland is positioned central to the globe as the suture is tied. Postoperative swelling is managed with topical antibiotic-corticosteroid preparations. Recurrence is uncommon and managed by reoperation.

F, An alternate, easier but less preferable technique involves placing a hemostat proximal to the portion of gland to be excised. *G,* Resection of gland distal to crushing. From Peiffer RL Jr et al: Surgery of the canine orbit, adnexa, and globe. Part V: Conjunctiva and Nictitating Membrane. *Companion Animal Practice* 1:15–28, November 1987.

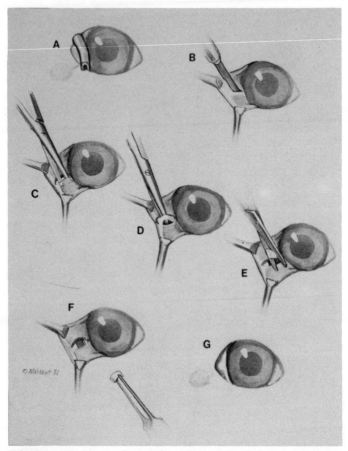

FIGURE 5-10. Repair of everted cartilage of the nictitating membrane. *A,* Appearance prior to surgery. *B,* Incision of mucosa on the bulbar surface of the nictitating membrane over the deformed cartilage. *C,* Blunt dissection with strabismus scissors to free the cartilage from the bulbar and palpebral mucosa. The cartilage is dissected free (*D*) and the deformed cartilage is resected (*E*). *F,* Mucosa may be sutured with knots buried or the incision left to heal by secondary intention. *G,* Immediately postoperatively the membrane should lie flat on the globe. Topical antibiotics and corticosteroids are dispersed postoperatively. From Peiffer RL Jr et al: Surgery of the canine orbit, adnexa, and globe. Part V: Conjunctiva and Nictitating Membrane. *Companion Animal Practice* 1:15–28, November 1987.

Immune-Mediated Hypertrophy (IMH)

IMH is characterized by focal thickening and/or depigmentation of the third eyelid. The condition may or may not be associated with chronic superficial keratitis (CSK or pannus). Pathogenesis involves infiltration of plasma cells and lymphocytes.

Like CSK, the cause of third eyelid IMH is not fully understood but has an immunological basis. The condition is exacerbated by ultraviolet light, with increased incidence in summer and high altitudes. Breed predisposition includes German Shepherds, Long-haired Dachshunds, Collie types, and Greyhounds. The condition is characterized by bilateral prominence of the third eyelid; close observation reveals diffuse thickening, with an irregular palpebral surface and a purple-pink coloration. Marginal depigmentation is not always present but is almost pathognomonic. Differentiations to consider include other causes of proliferative and follicular conjunctivitis. Conjunctival scrapings or biopsy confirm the diagnosis. Treatment is identical CSK; IMH of the third eyelid does not respond as dramatically or as readily as the corneal lesions. Topical corticosteroids on a regular (bid) basis, administered to effect in each individual patient, will generally provide satisfactory control.

Tumors

Tumors of the third eyelid may be inflammatory or neoplastic; the former group includes the immune-mediated granulomatous process seen most frequently in the Collie but which can affect any breed and present as a smooth pink nodule involving the cornea, conjunctiva, and/or palpebral surface of the third eyelid (Figure 5–11). These lesions are typically variably responsive to corticosteroids or azathioprine; treatment by excisional biopsy and local topical and/or subconjunctival corticosteroids is recommended, with systemic corticosteroids and/or azathioprine reserved for cases that cannot be controlled by this regimen.

The palpebral surface is uncommonly involved in neoplastic processes, with papillomas and hemangiomas most frequently encountered. Localized tumors are best removed by partial-thickness excision; small defects can be left to heal by second intention, larger defects apposed with 7-0 absorbable material. Adenocarcinomas of the third eyelid gland arise from the bulbar surface and need to be differentiated from prolapsed glands. The tumors are likely to be invasive at the base of the third eyelid, and the most effective treatment involves removal of the entire third eyelid with exploration of the inferior nasal orbit. The malignant nature of these tumors demands aggressive treatment, although removal of the third eyelid will predispose the eye to KCS and/or exposure keratoconjunctivitis.

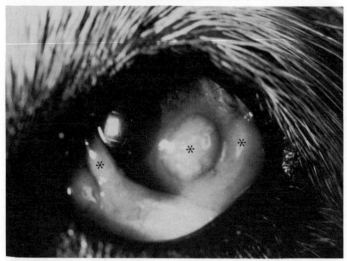

FIGURE 5-11. Immune-mediated proliferative keratoconjunctivitis in a 4-year-old female collie; lesions (∗) involve the limbus, cornea, and anterior surface of the third eyelid.

Bilateral Third Eyelid Protrusion in Cats

Bilateral protrusion of the third eyelid (haws) is a condition seen in young cats thought to be related to viral neuritis and subsequent sympathetic denervation of the third eyelid. The disease occurs frequently one to two weeks after a bout of upper respiratory or gastrointestinal inflammation and is painless and self-limiting, with resolution occurring over several weeks.

Other Causes of Protrusion of the Third Eyelid

A number of other conditions will result in protrusion of the third eyelid; unilateral prominence may be a feature of space-occupying orbital lesions (neoplasms and cellulitis), Horner's syndrome, dysautonomia, external irritative disorders (keratitis), symblepharon, or proliferative conjunctivitis. Protrusion due to orbital atrophy from general poor health and/or dehydration or previous myositis is bilateral. Thorough history and ophthalmic examination will generally allow specific diagnosis.

Pseudoprominence Related to Marginal Depigmentation

As a normal variant of pigmentation, animals may have marginal depigmentation of the leading edge of the third eyelid, which is usually pigmented. This condition gives an impression of prominence, especially if it is present unilaterally. The problem should be recognized as cosmetic rather than pathologic, and treatment is not required.

NASOLACRIMAL SYSTEM

As the signs of nasolacrimal obstruction, hypersecretion, or deficiency are manifested as ocular discharge, these conditions are discussed in detail in Chapter 7.

CORNEA AND SCLERA

Tumors

Tumors of the cornea are uncommon and may be divided into proliferative inflammatory disorders, choristomas, inclusion cysts, and neoplasmas.

Proliferative corneal inflammatory disease includes proliferative keratoconjunctivitis and chronic superficial keratitis in the dog and eosinophilic keratitis in the cat. The Collie is predisposed to proliferative keratoconjunctivitis, which may involve the cornea primarily or as a extension of a limbal lesion. Clinical appearance is that of an elevated, smooth, pink nodular lesion due to granulomatous, presumed immune-mediated inflammation (see Figure 5-11). Diagnosis should be confirmed by excisional biopsy; medical treatment with corticosteroids and/or azothioprine is required to prevent recurrence.

The cat is subject to eosinophilic keratitis, also felt to be an immune-mediated condition. The disease is usually unilateral and is characterized by a vascularized subepithelial corneal plaque, frequently with gray granules or flakes on its irregular surface (Figure 5-12). Lesions of eosinophilic dermatitis may but usually do not accompany it. Scrapings will demonstrate chronic inflammatory cells with numerous eosinophils and mast cells; excisional biopsy via lamellar keratectomy may be required to confirm the diagnosis. Topical and/or systemic corticosteroids or judicious use of megosterol acetate will cause regression of the lesion, and long-term treatment is frequently required for control.

Chronic superficial keratitis (CSK, pannus) may present initially because of abnormal appearance; the condition is discussed in detail in Chapter 4.

Corneal inclusion cysts present as elevated gray to yellow nodules on the corneal surface; previous trauma is the most likely cause. The condition is painless and managed with excision biopsy by lamellar keratotomy.

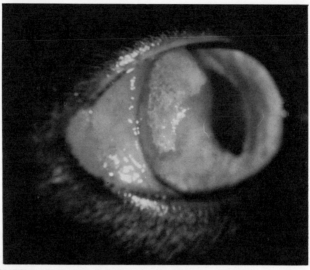

FIGURE 5-12. Eosinophilic keratitis in an 8-year-old Persian cat. Appearance may vary from the discrete leukoplakic lesion seen here to diffuse corneal involvement with granulation tissue.

Corneal dermoids are choristomatous tumors consisting of displaced epidermal tissue that may involve the conjunctiva and third eyelid, limbus, and/or cornea. The associated hairs result in irritation with blepharospasm and epiphora; excision by lamellar keratectomy and reconstruction (if necessary) is usually uncomplicated.

Squamous cell carcinoma of the cornea is an uncommon neoplasm in the dog and cat. The lesion appears leukoplakic (white plaque) because of keratin production by the neoplastic squames and may involve the cornea alone or be continuous with limbal and/or conjunctival involvement. Excisional biopsy via lamellar keratectomy is the treatment of choice.

The cornea may be involved secondarily in the extension of ocular tumors, including limbal melanocytomas, anterior uveal melanomas, ciliary body adenocarcinomas, and, in the cat, ocular sarcomas. Corneal infiltration and lymphosarcoma, especially in the cat, are not uncommon.

Scleral neoplasms are likewise uncommon; the sclera is more frequently involved by extension of intraocular tumors. An exception is the limbal melanocytoma, a benign lesion of limbal melanocytes. The condition occurs in dogs and cats of all breeds and ages; there is a preferential predisposition for the superior quadrant, and German Shepherds and Golden Retrievers have an exceptionally high incidence. The lesion presents as a discrete, well-defined subconjunctival nodule just posterior to the limbus (Figure 5–13); the tumors grow expansively over time and can become quite extensive. Intraocular extension can occur but usually late in the course of the disease. The tumor is benign in terms of its biological behavior, and early lamellar resection with cryosurgery of the base is frequently curative. More extensive cases may be managed by full-thickness corneoscleral grafts; if intraocular extension occurs with complications of glaucoma and uveitis, enucleation is recommended.

The most difficult clinical differentiation of these jet-black lesions is that of anterior uveal melanomas with trans-scleral extension; a small percentage of these tumors have malignant potential, and enucleation is the treatment of choice. Differentiating the two conditions can be achieved by gonioscopy in early cases; anterior uveal melanomas with trans-scleral extension invariably will show gonioscopic invasion of the iridocorneal angle as well as involvement of the iris and/or ciliary body. Such changes are seen only late in the course of corneoscleral limbal melanocytomas. If in

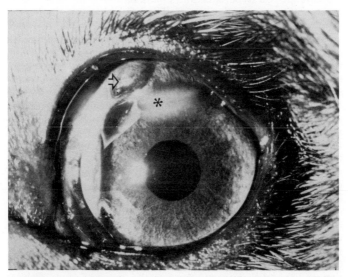

FIGURE 5–13. Limbal melanocytoma (*arrow*), left eye, in a young German Shepherd. Pigmentation may extend into the cornea and be characterized by a leading edge of edema and/or lipid degeneration (∘).

doubt, and the remaining eye is healthy, err on the conservative side and recommend enucleation. Transcleral extension of ciliary body adenocarcinomas is uncommon and generally more readily differentiated by their characteristic pink, fleshy, intraocular proliferations. Trans-sceral extension of feline ocular sarcomas generally appears as diffuse gray-pink proliferations.

Clinical differentiation of pigmented scleral tumors from congenital or acquired staphylomas must be made. These areas of outpouched thin sclera are generally located between the limbus and the equator, and because of the thin sclera the underlying uveal tissue gives the lesion a pigmented appearance. Congenital staphylomas are usually associated with multiple anomalies. Acquired lesions occur in association with chronic secondary glaucoma, and careful ophthalmic examination will usually reveal the distinction.

Episcleritis and/or scleritis is seen most commonly in the dog; the condition can be a challenging entity to diagnose clinically, and its proliferative form requires differentiation from neoplasia. Most cases tend to involve the anterior sclera, although posterior involvement occasionally is encountered, either associated with anterior episcleritis or as a distinct entity. The condition may be diffuse, in which case it is characterized by localized overlying conjunctival hyperemia and episcleral injection with a thick, meaty appearance to the episcleral tissues, or localized and nodular, in which case the lesions appear as discrete, pink, elevated, subconjunctival masses (Figure 5–14). In terms of etiopathogenesis, both forms are thought to represent immune-mediated processes against scleral collagen and are characterized histologically by granulomatous inflammation. These lesions are clinically similar to the proliferative keratoconjunctivitis seen in the Collie breed. Episcleritis and/or scleritis may be unilateral or bilateral, and any breed can be affected. In addition to the scleral involvement, uveitis and/or corneal edema may also be encountered. Posterior involvement may result in signs of a space-occupying orbital lesions including exophthalmos and an ophthalmoscopically evident chorioretinitis. Generally, the condition is not painful or accompanied by a prominent ocular discharge, the "red eye" being the primary presenting sign.

Diagnosis is based on clinical findings and biopsy of involved tissues if readily obtainable. Therapy involves the long-term administration of topical, subconjunctival, and/or systemic corticosteroids; cases nonresponsive to corticosteroids generally respond to azothioprine. As is generally the case in immune-mediated disease, steroid therapy is titered to the response of the disease and the particular patient in regard to frequency and duration of therapy.

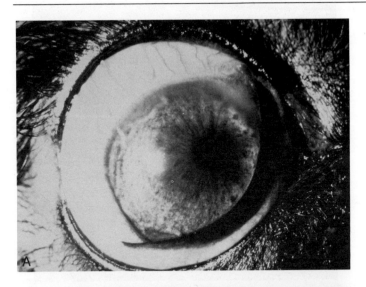

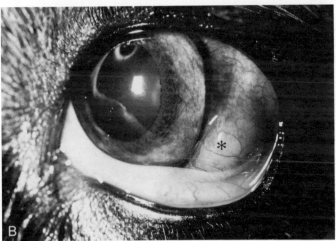

FIGURE 5-14. Immune-mediated scleritis. *A,* Diffuse anterior scleritis, right eye, of a 6-year-old Cockapoo. The episcleral and conjunctival vessels are engorged and there is corneal involvement superior nasally. *B,* Nodular anterior scleritis (∘) in a middle-aged mixed-breed canine.

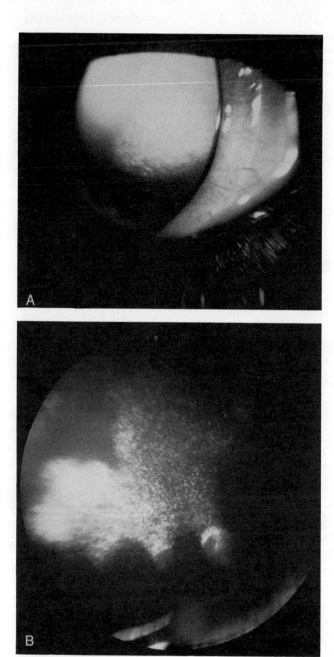

FIGURE 5-15. *See legend on the opposite page.*

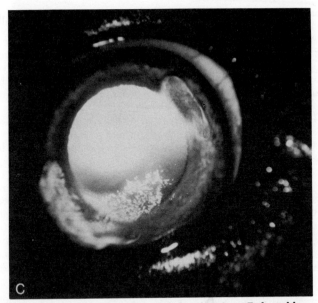

FIGURE 5-15. Lipid dystrophies and degenerations. Refractable crystalline subepithelial deposits are seen in an American Cocker Spaniel (*A*); at high magnification, in a 14-year-old Beagle (*B*); and a 5-year-old German Shepherd with hypothyroidism (*C*). Note the vascularization of the lesion in the last case.

Alterations in Corneal Transparency

Alterations in corneal transparency can be responsible for an abnormal appearance to the eye as well as visual impairment if extensive, and pain and discharge if inflammatory in nature. Such processes may involve the deposition of lipid, calcium, or other materials in the cornea; pigmentary keratitis as a consequence of chronic exposure and/or irritation; vascular and/or inflammatory infiltrate as part of an active inflammatory process; related to scar formation, usually as a sequela to inflammatory or traumatic processes; or involve the uptake of water by the corneal stroma, with resultant corneal edema.

Lipid and Calcific Dystrophics and Degenerations

The deposition of abnormal materials within the cornea may be a primary or secondary process. Primary corneal dystrophys are inherited, generally appear in the first few years of life, and manifest clinically as the deposition of fine, refractile, crystalline opacities within the corneal stroma, usually axially and frequently in a characteristic pattern for that particular disorder; for instance, the Siberian Husky typically has the material deposited in a circular fashion in the midperiphery, leaving a far peripheral and axial clear zone of cornea. The Golden Retriever has a corneal dystrophy that is manifested as a sausage-shaped or racetrack-type lesion. The condition is painless and generally not associated with significant visual impairment (Figure 5–15).

Lipid degenerations are nonspecific changes that are generally associated with chronic inflammation; they may be encountered in German Shepherds with chronic superficial keratitis or may be seen at the leading edge of limbal melanocytomas or inflammatory processes that have extended into the cornea. Lipid can be deposited secondary to hypercholesterolemia, the most common cause of which in the dog is hypothyroidism. This condition is encountered most frequently in the German Shepherd, and the lipid is deposited in an arcuate perilimbal fashion (see Figure 5–15). Calcium may be deposited in the cornea secondary to systemic metabolic diseases that result in hypercalcemia and/or hyperphosphatemia or as a complication of parotid duct transposition. These conditions can be associated with stubborn and persistent corneal ulcers in older dogs (Figure 5–16).

Treatment of lipid dystrophys and degenerations is seldom necessary; as mentioned, the epithelium over these lesions is usually intact and thus they are painless. Rarely are they dense enough to significantly affect functional vision, and animals seem to see very well through and around the deposits. Occasionally, the lipid will elicit an inflammatory response with superficial vascularization; if these conditions are nonresponsive to topical corticosteroids, lamellar keratectomy may be considered and is quite effective if the deposit is confined to the anterior stroma (and most of them are). Ulcers associated with calcific deposits tend not to heal unless the calcium is removed either by topical chelation with 1.0% EDTA or lamellar keratectomy.

Crystalline Keratopathy in the Dog and Cat

A self-limiting keratopathy associated with a deposition of crystalline material within the corneal stroma has been described in dogs and cats from the southeastern United States, notably Florida. The disease presents as single or multiple crystalline stromal opacities with indistinct margins and may be unilateral or bilateral. Frequently more than one animal in a particular household may be affected. The condition is painless and seldom extensive enough to affect vision; lamellar keratectomy may be performed in extensive cases. Noninflammatory infectious processes with fungi

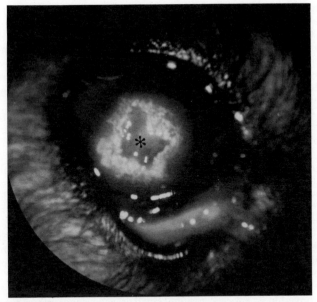

FIGURE 5-16. Calcific degeneration and associated ulceration (∘) in an old Miniature Poodle.

and/or acid fast bacilli, as well as noninfectious degenerative processes, have been speculated as the etiology.

Corneal Clouding Associated with Storage Disease

Diffuse corneal clouding in young animals may be one result of deposition of abnormal metabolic products related to inherited enzyme deficiencies. These conditions are rare in the dog and cat but should be suspected in the young animal presented with signs of diffuse, bilateral corneal clouding, visual impairment, and central nervous system signs.

Corneal Pigmentation

Pigmentation of the cornea may be associated with tear film deficiencies; chronic superficial keratitis; chronic exposure or irritation, common in the brachycephalic breeds; exposure associated with deficits of the fifth or seventh nerve; in the cat, related to a pigmentary stromal degeneration, most commonly referred to as a *corneal sequestrum* or *mummification,* or keratomycosis with a pigmented organism. All but the latter condition are discussed in detail elsewhere.

Corneal sequesterum is most likely an inherited disease in the cat, although multiple etiologies have been proposed. The condition can be seen in cats of virtually any age. Although any breed can be affected, the Persian and Siamese have the highest incidence. The condition may be unilateral or bilateral, the latter not always concurrently.

Clinically, the lesion appears as an axial or paraxial area of stromal discoloration that usually commences as a diffuse, golden-brown opacification. Over time, the lesion will progress to a discrete plaque of degenerative stromal tissue (Figure 5–17). While the epithelium overlying the lesion is intact, pain is usually minimal; occasional blepharospasm and epiphora may be noted. Invariably, the overlying epithelium ulcerates and the condition becomes more painful. Frequently, limbal corneal superficial vascularization to the lesion can be noted.

Treatment is by excision by lamellar keratectomy (Figure 5–18); the vast majority of lesions are localized within the anterior stroma and can be totally excised. If the excision is excessively deep, postoperative support with a nictitating flap is indicated. The lesions typically heal with mild scarring. If the lesion cannot be removed in its entirety, residual small areas of degenerative tissue may be reasonably tolerated, or progression may recur.

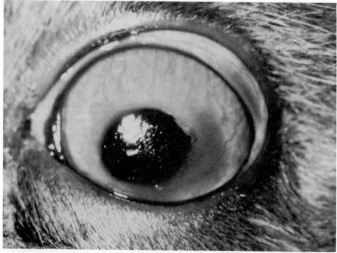

FIGURE 5–17. Corneal sequestrum in a young Persian cat.

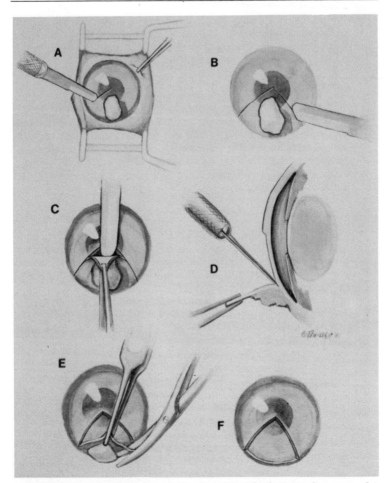

FIGURE 5-18. Lamellar keratectomy. *A* and *B*, The lesion to be removed is outlined with a scalpel blade to a depth of up to half the corneal thickness. *C* and *D*, The edge of the tissue to be excised is grasped with fine forceps, and lamellar dissection is performed with a scalpel blade, the blade edge parallel to the corneal surface. *E*, Once the dissection is carried to the limbus, the tissue is excised with scissors. From Peiffer RL Jr et al: Surgery of the canine and feline orbit, adnexa, and globe. Part VI: Surgery of the cornea. *Companion Animal Practice* 1:3–13, December 1987.

Pigment-producing fungi have been identified as corneal pathogens, and mycotic keratitis may present with a pigmented plaque. Diagnosis is made by corneal scraping. The condition is treated with topical antimycotic agents.

Keratitis

Corneal inflammation, either ulcerative or nonulcerative, is accompanied by edema and infiltration of the cornea by inflammatory cells acutely, blood vessels and granulation tissue if chronic, and scarring in resolving stages, all of which will contribute to give the eye an abnormal appearance. These conditions are generally associated with some degree of pain; keratitis is discussed detail in a later chapter.

Corneal Edema

Diffuse corneal edema will impart a hazy bluish opacification to the cornea that may be localized or diffuse, depending upon the severity and extent of the primary process. Corneal edema may occur secondary to active keratitis; secondary to intraocular disease, notably uveitis and glaucoma; as a result of blunt trauma to the eye; and as the result of a primary endothelial cell degeneration. The unifying feature of all of these processes is abnormal function of the corneal endothelium, which is essential for maintenance of relative stromal dehydration. When the endothelial cells, which have some regenerative capacity in the canine and very little in the cat, are significantly compromised, the corneal stroma takes on extracellular fluid with resultant swelling and opacification. If edema is severe, the fluid can accumulate into blisters that give the corneal epithelium an irregular contour; should these accumulations of fluid rupture, a painful, slow-healing ulceration will result.

One of the most dramatic examples of uveitis-associated corneal edema is the "blue eye" that occurs following infection with canine adenovirus or vaccination with the modified live virus. The virus has been demonstrated to localize within the corneal endothelium; as the body mounts an immune response, antigen-antibody complexes stimulate neutrophilic lysozymes, which damage the endothelium with resultant edema. The Afghan appears predisposed, and the condition may be unilateral or bilateral. The reaction typically occurs seven to fourteen days following vaccination. Generally, the corneal edema will resolve over time but may take many weeks. In this particular condition, secondary glaucoma is a not uncommon and generally challenging complication.

Corneal endothelial dystrophy occurs in older dogs, notably Boston Terriers, Chihuahuas, Dachshunds, and Miniature Poodles. Typically, the condition is bilateral and presents as a corneal edema that starts either in the temporal quadrants or axially (Figure 5–19). Over a period of months, the condition tends to be insidiously progressive. In the majority of affected dogs, the condition does not become clinically significant over the animal's remaining years. An occasional dog develops visual impairment due to the corneal edema and/or bullous keratopathy, with the formation of intracorneal bullae that rupture with resultant ulceration that tends to be both painful and persistent.

An inherited stromal dystrophy with edema as its primary manifestation has been described in the Manx cat, and acquired edema associated with extensive PPMs has been observed in the dog. Acute bullous keratopathy of undetermined etiology has been noted to occur spontaneously in the cat (Figure 5–20). Aberrant microfilaria in the anterior chamber of the canine can physically damage the endothelium with resultant edema.

Topical hyperosmotics are recommended therapy; the authors have not been impressed with their efficacy but prescribe them out of desperation. Third eyelid flaps are useful in stimulating ulcers to heal and supporting bullae. Permanent, thin conjunctival flaps will resolve edema and prevent bullous keratopathy with restoration of some vision (through the flap) in severe cases; corneal transplantation (penetrating keratoplasty) may likewise be contemplated in these patients. In general, cataract surgery is contraindicated in dogs with endothelial dystrophy.

Corneal Scarring

Congenital corneal opacification may be associated with congenital endothelial dystrophy or corneal attachments of persistent pupillary membranes. Congenital endothelial dystrophy is an uncommon condition seen in the American Cocker Spaniel as well as other breeds and appears as localized plaque of pigment and fibrous tissue on the axial endothelial surface. The condition appears to be nonprogressive, and treatment is not required. Likewise, corneal opacification associated with PPMs are stable and compatible with good vision. Superficial scarring in young pups and litters is a frequent result of ophthalmia neonatorium that will usually resolve with time.

Healing of corneal wounds results in disruption of normal lamellar architecture with an associated scar, the significance of which depends on the severity and location of the corneal wound; central scars in the pupillary axis are more likely to affect vision significantly compared to peripheral scars. Clinically, a corneal scar appears as a white, irregular opacity of an otherwise uninvolved cornea. Some remodeling and improvement usually occur over long periods of time; surgical excision of scar tissue with or without grafting is rarely indicated.

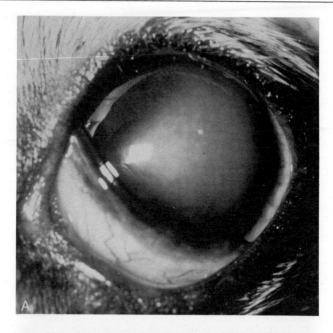

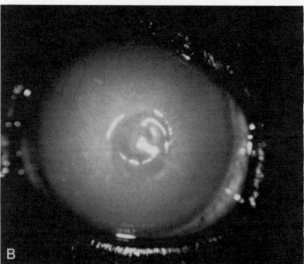

FIGURE 5-19. Corneal edema associated with endothelial cell dystrophy in an older Dachshund (*A*) and a Boston Terrier (*B*). A ruptured bulla has resulted in an axial ulcer in the terrier.

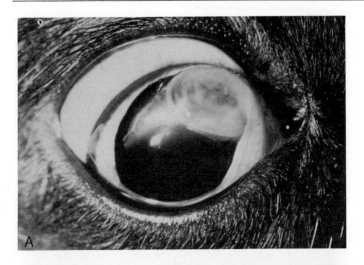

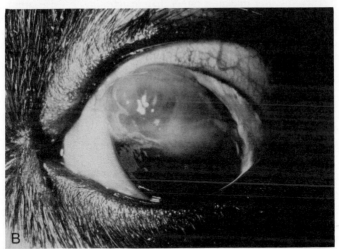

FIGURE 5-20. Acute idiopathic feline bullous keratopathy in a middle-aged domestic shorthair, right (A) and left (B) eye. The bullae are of acute onset in an intense normal eye, bilateral, and localized, with surrounding normal cornea, and involve only the anterior stroma. Nictitating membrane flaps assist healing, which results in mild scarring.

Corneoscleral Lacerations

Possibility of corneoscleral lacerations should be considered in any case of ocular or periocular trauma, especially in eyes with hyphema and low IOP. Although most will be readily evident as defects involving the limbus and cornea, the possibility of a more posterior defect should be kept in mind and explored if necessary. Typically, uveal tissue seals the defect and appears as an irregular, protruding, pigmented mass that may be covered with fibrin and/or hemorrhage.

These are ophthalmic emergencies that warrant prompt examination and repair with the patient under general anesthesia. Exposed and desiccated and/or obviously infected or contaminated extraocular tissue may be conservatively excised; cautery is helpful to minimize the usually vigorous hemorrhage that accompanies excision. Viable and healthy tissue may be reposited with a cyclodialysis spatula. Simple interrupted sutures of 7-0 smaller absorbable sutures for the cornea and 5-0 or smaller for the sclera are used to appose the wound; corneal sutures should be three-quarter thickness rather than penetrating. Intense antimicrobial and anti-inflammatory therapy is indicated. Prognosis is guarded and dependent on the extent of the original injury, with complications of corneal scarring, lens-induced uveitis, retinal detachment, endophthalmitis, and phthisis bulbi commonly encountered.

ANTERIOR SEGMENT

The anterior segment consists of all the ocular tissues anterior to the anterior hyaloid membrane (vitreous face) and thus in a strict sense includes the cornea, iris, ciliary body, iridocorneal angle, lens, and the anterior and posterior chambers. The chambers communicate through the pupil and contain the circulating aqueous. For our purposes, the cornea and lens are discussed separately. Critical examination of these tissues includes a focused beam of light (as available with the slitlamp) and magnification utilized in a darkened room.

Turbidity

The aqueous is normally a crystal clear fluid that appears optically empty with a focused light beam. If particulate matter is present, the beam of light is scattered and observable as it passes through the anterior chamber. Particulate matter in the aqueous may be protein (aqueous flare); white blood cells; red blood cells; neoplastic cells; or lipids. Clinically, aqueous turbidity requires distinction from corneal changes, notably edema. The conditions may coexist; if extensive corneal disease is present, critically examining the aqueous may be difficult.

Inflammation

Aqueous turbidity is most commonly caused by the products of inflammation—plasma proteins and inflammatory cells—that gain access via the iris and ciliary body vasculature, which become "leaky" in response to the chemical mediators of the inflammatory response. Pain is the most dramatic sign associated with anterior uveitis, due largely to spasm of the iridociliary musculature. However, the associated episcleral injection, corneal and iris edema, deep corneal vascularization, miotic pupil, and turbidity contribute to a markedly abnormally appearing eye! Neutrophils may settle out to the inferior quadrants to form a hypopyon. Protein may organize into a fibrin or fibrocellular clot. Intraocular pressure is low due to decreased production of aqueous. Anterior uveitis is not infrequently accompanied by posterior uveitis, and posterior segment examination is indicated.

If uveitis is chronic, pain less less likely to be the presenting sign and abnormal appearance more so. Flare is mild. Macrophages and lymphocytes tend to adhere to the corneal endothelium to form keratic precipitates (KPs). Iris changes include hyperpigmentation, inflammatory nodules, and dilation of iris vasculature. The cat may have feline nodular iritis (Figure 5-21), an interesting condition of undetermined etiology manifested by gray lymphoid follicles on the anterior iris surface. Although the condition is somewhat steroid responsive, secondary glaucoma is a frequent sequela. Immune-mediated uveitis may be accompanied by dermal depigmentation notably involving the muzzle or eyelids; this condition is suspected to be an autoimmunity against melanin.

Diagnosis is made upon presenting signs; in unilateral cases, careful scrutiny of the fellow eye is indicated. Symptomatic therapy (local and systemic broad-spectrum antibiotics, anti-inflammatory agents, and topical mydriatics) should be initiated while attempts to determine the etiology are pursued; these are summarized in Table 5-1. In all cases, thorough ophthalmic and physical examination is mandatory, and thoracic radiographs, hematology, serologic testing, and aqueouscentesis should be considered.

The keys to the appropriate management of the uveitis patient, then, are diagnosis, vigorous symptomatic treatment, and pursuit of the etiology. Medically uncontrollable lens-induced uveitis is an indication for lens removal. Immune-mediated cases may require chronic therapy with corticosteroids and/or azothioprine. Ultimate prognosis in anterior uveitis will depend upon cause and response to therapy.

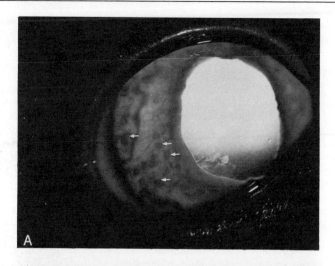

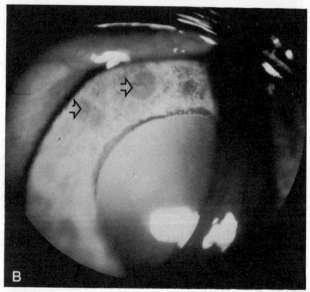

FIGURE 5–21. Feline nodular iritis in the right eye of a 4-year-old Siamese cat (*A*) and the right eye of a 10-year-old domestic shorthair (*B*). The iris nodules (*arrows*) are composed of lymphocytes. The condition may be unilateral or bilateral, not associated with systemic disease, and somewhat corticosteroid sensitive. Secondary glaucoma is not an uncommon sequela.

TABLE 5-1. Common Causes of Uveitis.

CANINE	FELINE	BOTH SPECIES
Brucellosis	FIP	Trauma
Systemic mycoses	Systemic mycoses	Keratitis
Ehrlichiosis	Toxoplasmosis	Lens-induced
		Septicemia
		Bacteremia
		Intraocular neoplasia
		Primary
		Secondary
		lymphosarcoma
		Immune-mediated
		(idiopathic)

Sequelae of anterior uveitis that may impart an abnormal appearance include:

1. Fibrinous adhesions that subsequently organize may form between the iris and anterior lens capsule (posterior synechiae) or corneal endothelium (anterior synechiae). These are generally permanent; the pupillary margin becomes irregular if involved. Anterior synechiae occurring at the iris base obstruct the angle, and secondary glaucoma may result if more than half of the angle is compromised. If adhesions form around the entire pupillary circumference, iris bombé results; aqueous cannot pass from the posterior to anterior chambers, the iris bulges forward, and secondary glaucoma results.

2. Secondary cataract (the composition of aqueous alters and disturbs nutrition to lens)

3. Iris and/or ciliary atrophy

4. Rubeosis iridis (iris neovascularization), which may lead to peripheral anterior synechiae and neovascular glaucoma and/or hyphema

5. Pupillary and cyclitic membranes (fibrovascular tissue) may form across the pupil and/or the anterior face of vitreous.

6. Phthisis bulbi

Aqueous Lipemia

Turbidity may also be caused by the presence of serum lipids in the aqueous. This condition is uncommon and thought to occur with concomitant uveitis and hyperlipemia. Common associations include spontaneous hyperlipoproteinemia, diabetes mellitus, pancreatitis, and hypothyroidism.

Clinical diagnosis is not difficult; onset is acute and the associated uveitis is usually mild. The diffuse pearly opaqueness of the aqueous is dense and more dramatic than flare and quite distinct from the fluffiness of hypopyon.

Initiate nonspecific uveitis therapy and pursue underlying primary causes. The condition will usually resolve over a period of days.

Hemorrhage (Hyphema)

Blood in the anterior segment may settle and form a distinct zone in the inferior anterior chamber or may be diffuse. The most likely causes include:

1. Trauma
2. Severe uveitis
3. Capillary fragility caused by toxemia/septicemia
4. Systemic clotting disorders associated with blood dyscrasias or toxicity
5. Iridal and/or retinal neovascularization
6. Retinal detachment and/or vitreous hemorrhage
7. Intraocular tumors, especially vascular tumors such as hemangiomas

Diagnosis of hyphema is self-evident (Figure 5–22); the chal-

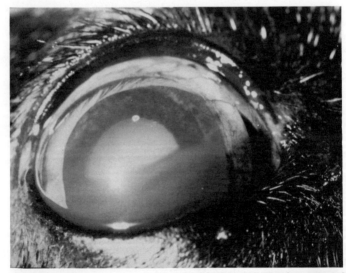

FIGURE 5–22. Spontaneous hyphema, right eye, in a Beagle associated with immune-mediated thrombocytopenia; mucous membrane petechiae were present.

lenge lies in determination of cause. The condition is usually unilateral unless an underlying systemic disorder exists; a thorough physical exam is indicated, with emphasis on mucous membranes for other sites of spontaneous hemorrhage. Examine the fellow eye for evidence of possible predisposing factors (such as Collie eye anomaly) and evaluate clotting by laboratory methods.

Treatment involves topical corticosteroids and mydriatics for the associated uveitis. Blood will usually resorb spontaneously in a few days unless bleeding is continuous; vigorous activity should be discouraged, and cage rest is advisable. Prognosis depends on the cause and, if traumatic, on extent of associated damage rather than therapy. Secondary glaucoma is an uncommon sequela in the dog and cat.

Iris Atrophy

Iris atrophy is a degenerative process seen more commonly in the dog than the cat and may involve the pupillary margin or the stroma. The condition may be inherited; the Miniature Poodle is predisposed to stromal atrophy.

Pupillary atrophy is identified by an irregular scalloped appearance to the pupillary margin, with the marginal defects occasionally spanned by threads of uveal tissue. If the sphincter muscle is extensively involved, pupillary constriction will be impaired. Stromal atrophy appears as partial- or full-thickness defect in the iris, giving a "swiss cheese" appearance; distinction from iris colobomata can be made by history (Figure 5-23). Depending on involvement of the dilator and sphincter muscles, pupillary responses are variably impaired.

Iris atrophy is asymptomatic and requires no therapy; recognition is important, however, to allow critical interpretation of the PLR and other pupillary abnormalities.

Neoplasia

Both primary and secondary neoplasms may affect the anterior segment; most primary uveal tumors in animals involve the anterior uvea rather than the choroid.

Pigmented tumors are the most common primary intraocular tumor in both dog and cat, but clinical presentation and biological behavior is quite different between the species. In the dog, the majority are benign pigmented proliferations that involve the iris and ciliary body; choroidal melanomas occur but are quite rare. They may be benign, slow-growing, distinct iris lesions composed of normal or neoplastic melanocytes; the former are referred to as *freckles* and the latter as *nevi*. Canine uveal melanomas (Figure 5-24) may grow expansively into the anterior

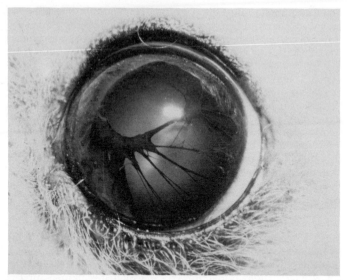

FIGURE 5–23. Iris stromal atrophy in an elderly Miniature Poodle, left eye.

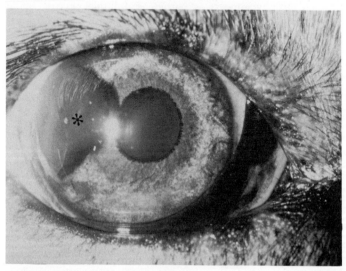

FIGURE 5–24. Anterior uveal melanoma (∘), right eye, in a 6-year-old German Shepherd–Collie mixed-breed dog.

and posterior chambers, posteriorly into the choroid, or through the limbal sclera, where they present as pigmented episcleral nodules. They may also be recognized as changes in iris pigmentation or by secondary processes including uveitis, glaucoma, and hyphema. A good rule of thumb is to suspect all cases of spontaneous unilateral uveitis, hyphema, and glaucoma (especially in breeds not genetically predisposed) as possible intraocular neoplasms until proven otherwise. Histologically, the majority are benign melanocytomas. Because a small percentage of canine uveal melanomas are malignant, enucleation is indicated in all animals with large, rapidly growing tumors, or melanomas complicated by uveitis and/or glaucoma.

Prognosis for overall health is generally favorable, but *always* do a thorough preoperative workup (we recommend a chest radiography and laboratory panel on all patients) and submit the globe to a pathologist; mitotic index is the best prognosticator of canine uveal melanomas.

Freckles and nevi occur in cats as well; although neoplastic transformation of these benign lesions has not been documented, they should be followed closely at regular intervals. Melanomas of the anterior uvea in cats usually involve the iris primarily and arise as diffuse rather than nodular proliferations. Secondary glaucoma and uveitis may occur. In contrast to dogs, these neoplasms tend to metastasize early, and high clinical suspicion is an indication for enucleation. As with the dog, a thorough preoperative workup is indicated. Prognosis is guarded, with metastatic disease noted months to years following surgery.

Ciliary body epithelial neoplasms are the second most common primary intraocular tumors in the dog and probably in the cat as well, although they are much less common in the feline. Although a rare undifferentiated variant (medulloepitheliomas) may be seen in young animals, these neoplasms typically are seen in middle-aged or older patients. They present as pigmented or, more frequently, nonpigmented pink proliferations; adenomas tend to grow between the anterior lens and posterior iris and can be observed through the pupil. Adenocarcinomas invade the iris base, appear as nonpigmented iris tumors, and may cause secondary glaucoma due to invasion and obliteration of the outflow pathways (Figure 5–25). As with melanomas, uveitis and intraocular hemorrhage can also occur secondary to these neoplasms. In the dog about fifty percent of ciliary body epithelial tumors will be benign and fifty percent malignant; in the cat, the majority of these tumors are malignant neoplasms. Enucleation is the treatment of choice; potential metastatic disease should be a consideration if the histopathology demonstrates a malignant tumor. We recommend a thorough physical examination and thoracic ra-

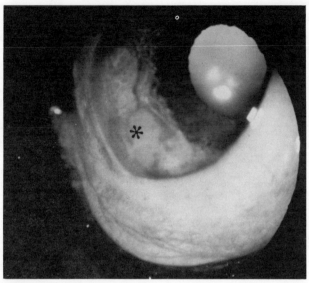

FIGURE 5-25. Ciliary body adenocarcinoma presenting as a nonpigmented proliferative lesion (∘) at the base of the iris, right eye, in a Brittany Spaniel.

diographs at the time of diagnosis and at three months following surgery.

Primary ocular sarcomas in the cat occur spontaneously or may be associated with previous trauma or inflammation, not unusually occurring several months to years prior to presentation. They may arise in either visual or blind phthisical globes, presumably from the uveal tissues. They appear as solid gray proliferations and are quite aggressive in terms of both extraocular extension and distant metastases. If suspected, preoperative evaluation should include skull and thoracic radiographs prior to enucleation; prognosis should be guarded. Because of the nature of this tumor, enucleation of blind phthisical feline eyes is indicated.

Other primary tumors that are uncommon have similar signs: a space-occupying ocular lesion with or without secondary uveitis, glaucoma, and/or intraocular hemorrhage. Neoplasia metastatic to the globe is likely to have similar presentation with a predisposition for the choroid; although lymphosarcoma is the most common secondary intraocular tumor, virtually any malignancy can involve the ocular tissues. Diagnosis depends upon maintaining a level of awareness of these diseases, the basic principle of looking beyond the eye with a thorough systemic evaluation, and, if indicated, confirmation by enucleation.

Differential diagnosis of primary or secondary intraocular neoplasia includes benign iris or ciliary body cysts; iris hyperpigmentation due to chronic uveitis; granulomatous inflammation, usually associated with the systemic mycoses; and other causes of uveitis, glaucoma, and intraocular hemorrhage.

Iris and Ciliary Body Cysts

Cysts of the iris and ciliary body epithelium may arise spontaneously or occur secondary to trauma or inflammation; they may be single or multiple, unilateral or bilateral, and adherent to the uvea (usually at the ciliary processes or pupillary margin) or free-floating in the anterior chamber. Certain breeds, notably the Boston Terrier and the Golden and Labrador Retrievers, are predisposed. These lesions are identifiable by their distinct round to oval shape and ability to transilluminate (Figure 5–26); an occasional ciliary body adenoma will be cystic but will not transilluminate as readily as a ciliary body cyst. Treatment is usually not necessary; if large or multiple cysts interfere with visual function, they can be readily aspirated.

LENS

Diseases of the lens can be subdivided into three broad groups: normal aging changes, or nuclear sclerosis; opacification, or cataract; and lens dislocation, all of which contribute to an altered appearance. Cataracts are frequently presented with accompanying visual impairment, and the glaucoma that accompanies lens dislocation brings both pain and visual impairment, as well as abnormal appearance; these conditions are discussed in detail elsewhere. This section will deal with those changes of the lens that are primarily manifested by abnormal appearance rather than visual impairment.

Cataracts may be presented with a complaint of abnormal appearance rather than visual impairment if the cataract is unilateral, with the animal compensating with the visual fellow eye, or if the cataract is incipient or immature, allowing the animal reasonable functional vision around or through the lens opacification.

Nuclear Sclerosis

Nuclear sclerosis is a normal aging change seen in dogs older than six or seven and in cats a bit later, usually not before age twelve. It is a result of hardening of the lens related to compression of central lens fibers, which continue to proliferate throughout life within the limited confines of the lens capsule. In older

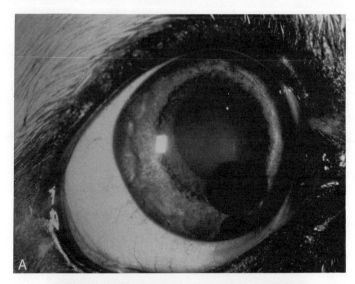

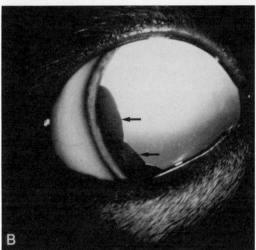

FIGURE 5-26. Iris (*A*) and ciliary body (*B, arrow*) cysts in a Golden Retriever and Siamese cat, respectively.

animals it is responsible for a change in the reflection through the pupil, from one that is black and shiny in the young dog or cat to one that is bluish and lusterless in the older animal. Although some degree of visual impairment accompanies nuclear sclerosis, it is by itself not a cause of significant visual loss, and affected animals get around quite well. Upon dilation of the pupil, nuclear sclerosis can be identified by its distinct margins within the center of the lens and by the ability to visualize a fundus reflex through the sclerotic nucleus; with a cataract, a fundus reflex cannot be observed. Nuclear sclerosis may be accompanied by cataractous change involving either the nucleus or the cortex; typically, senile cortical cataracts are *cuneiform*, that is, wedge-shaped or triangular, with the base at the equator. Senile cataracts progress slowly and rarely reach the point where functional vision is significantly affected.

Cataract

As discussed in the preceding chapter, the majority of cataracts in the canine are inherited and may be congenital or acquired; the specific features (location and biological behavior) of cataract in a particular breed are predictable and particular to that breed. Cataracts may be congenital and not inherited, such as those associated with lenticular attachments of persistent pupillary membranes, anterior or posterior suture lines, pigmented flecks on the anterior lens capsule, nuclear flecks and irregularities, and posterior capsular opacities associated with a persistent hyaloid artery or tunica vasculosa lentis, with or without persistent hyperplastic primary vitreous. Cataracts may be secondary, occurring associated with other ocular or systemic diseases; most common secondary causes are trauma, uveitis, and retinal atrophy in regard to ocular disease, and diabetes mellitus in regard to systemic diseases.

The diagnosis of cataract, then, warrants a thorough history, general physical, and ophthalmic examination in an attempt to define etiology and render a prognosis.

Lens Dislocation

Dislocated lenses may present because of abnormal appearance, although more frequently as associated signs of secondary glaucoma and/or uveitis that are more obvious to the client. Lens dislocation may be primary or secondary, complete or partial, and anterior or posterior. Primary lens luxations are most commonly encountered in the Terrier breeds and thought to be related to inherent weakness of the zonules. Secondary lens luxation may occur secondary to blunt or penetrating trauma or to chronic glaucoma with buphthalmos, where enlarging of the eye causes stretching of the zonules to the point of weakness. In some cases, determining whether the lens luxation was primary and the glaucoma secondary or vice versa may be difficult; probably the breed affected will provide the most conclusive evidence in this regard. For instance, Cocker Spaniels and Basset Hounds, which are predisposed to primary glaucoma, would likely be categorized in the latter group. Luxated lenses may be clear or cataractous; most lenses that have been dislocated for some time will become cataractous secondarily, and a clear luxated lens is usually indicative of a relatively short-term process. Mature cataractous lenses may likewise dislocate, sometimes with restoration of vision if the luxation is posterior and glaucoma does not develop. The duration, extent, and position of lens dislocation are critical in management.

Anterior lens luxations are identified by the presence of the lens in the anterior chamber; the most readily evident feature clinically is obscuration of the pupillary margin and observing the iris surface going behind the anteriorly luxated lens (Figure 5–27, *A*). The hallmarks of posterior luxation or subluxation are the presence of an aphakic crescent if the luxation is partial (Figure 5–27,*B*); in addition, the unsupported iris will tremble when the eye is moved (iridodonesis). With total luxation, the lens can be visualized lying on the floor of the vitreous cavity.

Anterior lens luxation should be regarded as ophthalmic emergencies; secondary glaucoma is bound to occur sooner or later, and prompt removal of the luxated lens is in most cases curative. If the pressure is elevated, it should be managed with intravenous mannitol and other hypotensive agents and the case referred to a specialist for intracapsular extraction. Time is of the essence in preserving vision in these eyes! Posteriorly luxated or subluxated lenses should be removed if the eye is potentially visual and if there are clinical signs of uveitis and/or glaucoma associated with the condition. Posteriorly luxated or subluxated lenses without other signs may be managed conservatively, provided that they can be followed closely. Topical 2% pilocarpine will assist in keeping the pupil constricted and the lens in the posterior chamber, where it is less likely to cause significant acute problems.

Primary lens luxation is a bilateral disease; the fellow eye in such cases should have a thorough dilated examination, including gonioscopy. Fellow eyes in such cases are at risk for future involvement.

POSTERIOR SEGMENT

Leukocoria

Leukocoria means "white pupil"; the most common causes in the dog and cat are cataract, a persistent hyperplastic primary vitreous and/or persistent tunica vasculosa lentis, vitritis, and reti-

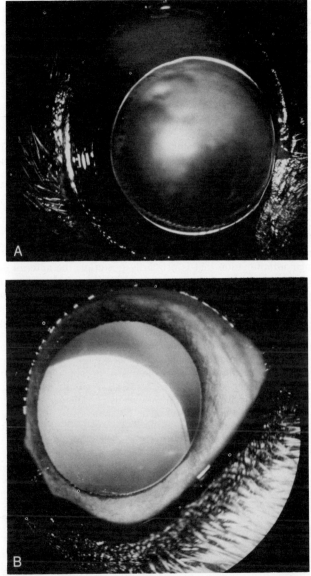

FIGURE 5-27. Anterior lens luxation (A) in the right eye of a 7-year-old Terrier and posterior subluxation (B) in a Siberian Husky, left eye.

nal detachment. Less commonly, a neoplastic process, such as a nonpigmented ciliary body tumor or posterior segment neoplasm, may show such a clinical appearance. Depending upon the severity and cause of the problem, visual impairment and/or signs of uveitis may accompany it. Leukocoria is a nonspecific diagnosis, the presence of which demands further pursuit with thorough ophthalmic examination.

Vitreous Inflammatory Infiltrate

The vitreous is essentially a hydrated collagenous gel that is avascular; tissue elements that encroach upon the vitreous commonly come from the retina and/or ciliary body vasculature. Thus, *vitritis* is strictly speaking a misnomer, as the vitreous becomes inflamed only secondarily to primary inflammation of adjacent tissues. Vitritis may be present but difficult to diagnose if the anterior segment is involved in the inflammatory process, simply because of decreased visibility due to anterior segment changes including corneal edema, aqueous cell and flare, and miosis. With ocular inflammation that is primarily posterior, the anterior segment may be only subtly involved, with mild episcleral injection and slight flare; in these cases, iris involvement may be minimal and the pupil may be normal in size. The vitreous in these cases is hazy, and retinal detail is difficult to visualize by ophthalmoscope. Frequently, inflammatory cells adhere to the posterior lens capsule. Vitritis may be exogenous, resulting from bacteria or fungi introduced by penetrating injury, or endogenous, from systemic infectious or ocular disease. Etiologies to be considered include feline infectious peritonitis, toxoplasmosis, systemic mycosis, and bacteremia. Rupture of the posterior lens capsule can cause vitritis. If a specific diagnosis cannot be determined by physical and laboratory examination, aspiration of vitreous with vitreous cytology and culture may be helpful in defining the etiology of the problem.

Treatment and prognosis will depend upon the cause; sequelae of vitritis include vitreous abscess and the formation of vitreous traction bands, with tractional retinal detachment.

Vitreous Hemorrhage

Vitreous hemorrhage is most frequently the result of bleeding from the retina; it may occur secondary to systemic clotting disorders or from trauma. It may be a manifestation of systemic disease, notably hypertensive oculopathy, which in the dog and cat is most frequently associated with chronic renal disease, or it may be secondary to ocular disease, including retinal detachment, most frequently associated with preretinal neovascularization. In young animals, the condition may be associated with persistent hyaloid vessels and/or persistent hyperplastic primary vitreous. Some cases are idiopathic in that no cause can be determined.

Ultimate prognosis depends upon cause; idiopathic hemorrhages will resorb over several weeks, generally without significant sequelae. However, organizing hemorrhage may lead to vitreous traction bands and secondary retinal detachment. Thorough examination of the fellow eye and a complete physical examination is indicated.

Asteroid Hyalosis

This condition is not uncommonly seen in older dogs and is identified by tiny white refractile bodies, usually composed of calcium salts and cholesterol, suspended within formed vitreous (Figure 5-28). The condition is generally a nonspecific degenera-

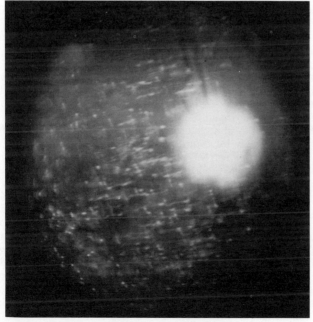

FIGURE 5-28. Asteroid hyalosis in an elderly Poodle.

tion seen in elderly patients; an association exists between asteroid hyalosis and ciliary body epithelial neoplasia. No treatment is necessary, as generally reasonable vision is maintained even through the densest asteroid accumulations.

Retinal Detachment

Retinal detachment is relatively uncommon in the dog and cat; generally, the presenting signs are those of visual impairment, although unilateral cases may go undetected due to compensatory unilateral vision in a particular animal; the preceding chapter discusses retinal detachment in detail. The majority of cases in dogs and cats are exudative or inflammatory retinal detachments occurring secondary to chorioretinitis or hypertensive oculopathy. Other causes include rhegmatogenous detachments and vitreous tractional detachments. The former are associated with retinal tears or holes and are most commonly seen in animals with Collie eye anomaly, which is associated with large peripheral tears (dialyses) or with atrophic retinal holes resulting from chorioretinitis. In relatively acute cases, pupillary light reflexes are intact, although the PLR deteriorates over time. Focal retinal detachments are identified as bullous elevations off the choroid-RPE surface; following the blood vessels along ophthalmoscopically is frequently the most reliable means of detection. In total retinal detachments, the retina presents a morning glory appearance as a gray, vascularized, retrolental membrane.

Prognosis is dependent upon cause and duration; following retinal detachment, photoreceptor degeneration occurs rather rapidly as the rods and cones are cut off from their nutritional supply from the choriocapillaris and the retinal pigment epithelium.

History is helpful in determination of cause. Congenital retinal detachments may be seen in the Collie or with retinal dysplasia in the Bedlington Terrier, English Springer Spaniel, or Labrador Retriever. Diastolic blood pressure should be determined to rule out hypertensive oculopathy in both dogs and cats; this condition is frequently, but not always, accompanied by intraocular hemorrhage. The most common cause of exudative retinal detachments in the cat is feline infectious peritonitis and systemic mycotic diseases in the dog. However, other infectious agents, including *Cryptococcus* and *Histoplasma* in the cat and *Brucella* and *Ehrlichia* in the dog, should be considered. Exudative detachments frequently accompany immune-mediated chorioditis, notably in the Akita. Primary or secondary intraocular neoplasia can also be associated with retinal detachments, notably feline lymphosarcoma.

Prognosis is dependent upon cause and duration; after several weeks, it is unlikely that the return of functional vision will occur, even if the retina is reattached. Exudative detachments will reattach if the inflammation is managed by treating the etiologic agent specifically as well as by nonspecific corticosteroid therapy. With detachments associated with hypertensive oculopathy, control of the high blood pressure will lead to reattachment; this is accomplished by control of dietary intake of salt, diuretics, and vasodilating drugs.

6 Orbital or Ocular Pain

Cynthia S. Cook

The recognition of ocular pain is often the first indication to the pet owner that an ophthalmic condition exists that requires veterinary attention. In domestic animals, the manifestations of discomfort associated with the eyes may be as variable as the temperaments of the animals themselves. Discharge, blepharospasm, protrusion of the third eyelid, photophobia, and pawing at the face are seen in acutely painful conditions. Among more stoic animals and in conditions with moderate discomfort, such as chronic glaucoma or uveitis, these symptoms may be less obvious with only mild depression, restlessness, and/or inappetence apparent to the owner.

ORBITAL CELLULITIS

Orbital cellulitis may be unilateral or bilateral and may rarely be accompanied by vision loss. The condition is caused by inflammation within the orbit resulting in acute exophthalmos and protrusion of the third eyelid with or without deviation of the globe (Figure 6-1). Pain is elicited upon opening the jaw, which compresses the orbital space. Resistance accompanied by pain is encountered upon attempts to digitally retropulse the globe (through closed eyelids) into the orbit. An occasional case fistulates to the conjunctival surface and presents with profuse purulent exudation; examination and probing under general anesthesia reveal the draining tract. Animals with orbital cellulitis are usually febrile and have an elevated white blood cell count with a left shift. The major differential diagnosis for exophthalmos is orbital neoplasia, which generally has a history of a slowly progressive condition and is not characterized by ocular pain. Chemosis is often present in cases of orbital cellulitis and may contribute to the initial impression that the globe itself is enlarged. Thus, this condition must be differentiated from glaucoma based on critical evaluation of the size of the globe (through comparison with the opposite eye, if unaffected) and by measurement of intraocular

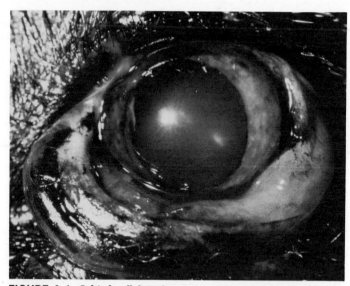

FIGURE 6-1. Orbital cellulitis demonstrating exophthalmos, chemosis, and protrusion of the third eyelid. The pupillary dilation may be an indication of optic nerve involvement.

pressure. If the optic nerve is uninvolved, pupillary light responses are normal, further distinguishing this condition from glaucoma.

The etiology in cases of orbital cellulitis often remains obscure. Suppurative conditions of the maxillary or frontal sinuses may extend to involve the orbit. Foreign body migration from the oral cavity or conjunctiva is often implicated but seldom confirmed. Inflammation of the zygomatic salivary gland may extend to involve the orbit. Examination of the oral mucosa behind the last upper molar on the affected side often reveals localized inflammation and occasionally purulent drainage. Aspiration by inserting a needle from the oral cavity into the orbit is often diagnostic; establishment of drainage into the mouth at this site may be therapeutic. The oral mucosa is incised and the underlying tissues bluntly dissected with a hemostat. Systemic treatment with broad-spectrum antibiotics (ampicillin is our drug of choice) usually provides resolution of the condition within five to seven days; medication should be continued for two weeks. Exophthalmos may lead to impaired blinking, and the cornea should be evaluated for evidence of exposure keratitis. Topical treatment with antibiotic ointment is of value to protect the cornea. If the corneal epithelium is intact, a topical ointment that contains a corticosteroid may reduce the conjunctival inflammation.

KERATITIS

Corneal Ulcers

Painful conditions involving the cornea are the most common ocular presentation for the general veterinary practitioner. Typically, these cases exhibit epiphora, blepharospasm, retraction of the globe, and protrusion of the third eyelid. Most cases of severe, acute corneal pain are associated with a corneal ulcer or laceration. Ulcerative keratitis may be caused by a single traumatic event, such as a cat scratch, or by a more insidious form of mechanical irritation related to eyelid abnormalities or a conjunctival foreign body. Evaluation of such cases is facilitated by the application of a topical anesthetic. Fluorescein staining to identify the extent and location of the corneal epithelial defect may give an indication of the source of the injury, particularly if eyelid conformation is at fault or a foreign body is present.

A diagnostic approach to ulcerative keratitis should involve a careful evaluation of the depth and extent of the defect and the detection of complicating factors such as infection or continued mechanical irritation from a foreign body or eyelid abnormalities. Corneal ulcers can be classified as *superficial,* involving only the epithelium and superficial stroma, or *deep,* extending into the deep stroma up to Descemet's membrane (Figure 6–2). In all cases of ulcerative keratitis, the conjunctival sac, particularly behind the third eyelid, should be examined under topical anesthesia for the presence of a foreign body. Traumatic, full-thickness corneal lacerations are best managed by direct suturing of the wound edges. Immediate repair (ideally with the use of an operating microscope) with fine, nonreactive suture material (nylon, 7-0 or smaller) often results in the preservation of visual function in eyes that might otherwise be lost. Corneal foreign bodies should be removed; surgical excision (keratectomy) of deeply embedded material may be necessary. The resultant ulcer should then be treated according to its depth and extent as described below.

Superficial corneal ulcers that are acute and accompanied by only a clear ocular discharge are usually managed easily with prophylactic application of a topical triple-antibiotic solution (neomycin, bacitracin, and polymyxin) twice daily until the animal is reexamined in seven to ten days and the eye found to be fluorescein-negative. Atropine solution is usually unnecessary in such cases and may actually impair reepithelialization by decreasing tear production. Recurrent epithelial erosions (indolent ulcers) present a unique type of superficial corneal ulceration that is slow to heal, often recurs, and is characterized by an edge of loose epithelium surrounding the fluorescein-positive defect (Figure 6–3). These are seen most often in the Boxer breed, although

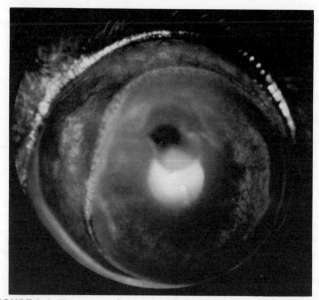

FIGURE 6–2. Deep corneal ulcer extending centrally to Descemet's membrane. The adjacent cornea is edematous; however, Descemet's membrane remains clear. This ulcer should be managed using a conjunctival flap.

older dogs of any breed may be affected. Recurrent epithelial erosions are thought to be due to an abnormality in the adhesive qualities of the epithelial basement membrane. Removal of the nonadherent adjacent epithelium by careful debridement under topical anesthesia may be therapeutic. This procedure often needs to be repeated every seven to ten days and is followed by slow resolution over several weeks; prophylactic topical antibiotics should be used twice daily. In particularly chronic cases, a superficial keratectomy (removing the involved and adjacent epithelium, basement membrane, and superficial stroma) with the use of an operating microscope may be required. The use of a 20-gauge needle to pattern multiple superficial punctate keratotomies of the ulcer base has recently been shown to stimulate resolution of some cases of recurrent epithelial erosions.

Corneal ulcers that are accompanied by a mucopurulent ocular discharge and/or evidence of chronicity (pigmentation, vascularization, scarring) require more careful evaluation of eyelid con-

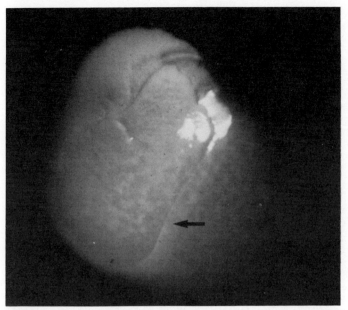

FIGURE 6-3. A superficial corneal ulcer typical of a recurrent epithelial erosion (Boxer ulcer). The elevated epithelial edge (*arrow*) is characteristic of this basement membrane defect. Repeated debridement is often necessary to resolve these ulcers.

formation and tear production. A Schirmer tear test is indicated in these cases.

Deep corneal ulcers and descemetoceles require more aggressive management. As with the superficial lesions, identification of the etiology of the injury should be made if possible. A Schirmer tear test and culture of the defect should be routinely performed. For deep ulcers, mechanical support is of value to prevent perforation. A third eyelid flap should be used in cases where the defect is no more than half the corneal thickness and does not appear to be infected. The procedure is performed under light general anesthesia using two or three mattress sutures and stents to attach the third eyelid to the upper conjunctival fornix (Figure 6-4). For deeper ulcers or descemetoceles, filling the defect with healthy tissue through the use of a conjunctival graft is indicated. A 360° conjunctival flap sutured with three to four mattress sutures is the easiest to perform (Figure 6-5). The sutures are removed in ten to fourteen days and the conjunctiva allowed to slowly

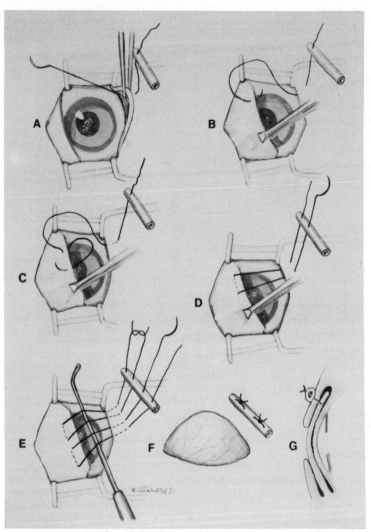

FIGURE 6–4. Eyelid-sutured third eyelid. *A,* The upper lid is grasped, and a suture is placed through the superior temporal lid into the fornix. *B,* The suture is then passed beneath the arms of the cartilage or through the base of the cartilage at the midpoint. *C,* Note direction of the needle in placing the mattress suture. *D,* The first suture placed. *E,* The second suture is placed in a similar fashion; sutures may be placed through or over a stent to minimize tension. *F,* Completion of third eyelid. Topical medication may be applied to the flap surface. *G,* Cross-section demonstrates proper positioning of sutures and third eyelid. From Peiffer RL Jr et al: Surgery of the canine and feline orbit, adnexa, and globe. Part V: Conjunctiva and nictitating membrane. *Companion Animal Practice* 1:15–28, 1987.

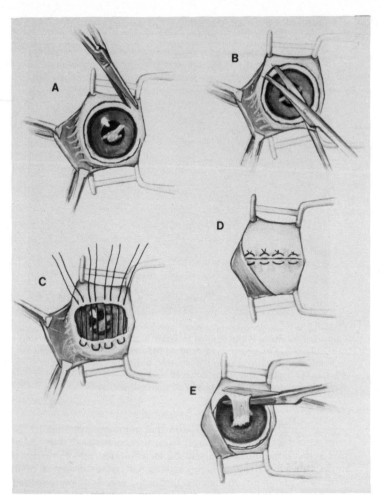

FIGURE 6-5. Fornix-based 360° conjunctival flap. Scissors are used to sharply incise (*A*) and bluntly dissect beneath (*B*) the perilimbal conjunctiva. Retraction of the nictitating membrane facilitates the dissection, which should be extended to the fornix so that the conjunctiva is freely mobile. Everting mattress sutures of 4-0 silk are placed and snugly secured (*D*); use of an overlying nictitating membrane flap is optional. Topical medication may be applied to the flap surface. After 10 to 14 days, the sutures are removed under topical anesthesia and the conjunctiva is allowed to retract. The grafted tissue may be separated by sliding a small blunt scissors between the cornea and bridge of conjunctiva and incising the tissue (*E*). The adherent portion of conjunctiva may be left to be extruded or incorporated into the corneal scar. From Peiffer RL Jr et al: Surgery of the canine and feline orbit, adnexa, and globe. Part V: Conjunctiva and nictitating membrane. *Companion Animal Practice* 1:15–28, 1987.

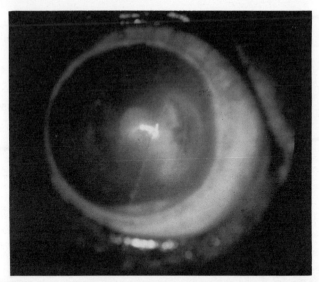

FIGURE 6-6. A deep corneal ulcer complicated by bacterial infection. Compare the dense white stromal infiltrate in this eye to the simple edema in Figure 6-2. The presence of exudate (neutrophils) ventrally within the anterior chamber (hypopyon) is another indication that this is a septic process. This ulcer should be cultured and managed with a conjunctival flap, topical atropine, and topical and systemic antibiotics.

recede back into position. Tissue that remains adherent to the corneal defect may be severed from its conjunctival attachment under local anesthesia and will be incorporated into the corneal scar or slowly extruded. Deep lesions that are extensive in area, with or without infectious complications, may best be managed by other surgical procedures, including corneoscleral transposition, and are best referred to a veterinary ophthalmologist. Deep corneal ulcers should initially be treated with topical antibiotic solution (neomycin, bacitracin, and polymyxin) four to six times daily, pending culture results. Atropine solution (twice daily) is of value in such cases to prevent iridocorneal adhesion should perforation occur and to treat the secondary uveitis that frequently accompanies deep corneal ulcers. Appropriate systemic antibiotics are also indicated.

Infectious processes may be a cause of ulcerative keratitis or, more commonly, a secondary complication. Corneal ulcers accompanied by a purulent discharge and/or corneal infiltrate or those that are refractory to treatment should arouse suspicion of an infectious component. Successful management is dependent upon establishment of an accurate diagnosis and intensive specific and antimicrobial therapy; the value of cytology and culture cannot be overemphasized. Scraping of the cornea under topical anesthesia can be used to obtain samples for cytology and culture. A slide may be prepared for cytologic evaluation using Gram's or Wright's stain to provide immediate information about the presence and type of bacterial or fungal infection. Bacterial keratitis may have a variable presentation, from a slowly advancing ulcer accompanied by stromal infiltrate (Figure 6-6) to one that progresses to perforation within hours. The presence of hypopyon (purulent exudate within the anterior chamber) as seen in Figure 6-6 is nearly always an indication of a septic process. Viral conditions such as herpesvirus most often present as a superficial, persistent corneal erosion with minimal discharge or infiltrate (Figure 6-7). If viral keratitis is suspected, a slide prepared from a corneal scraping can be submitted for immunologic diagnosis of herpesvirus. Fungal keratitis is usually associated with intense but localized corneal infiltrate (Figure 6-8).

Congenital conditions that may be accompanied by ulcera-

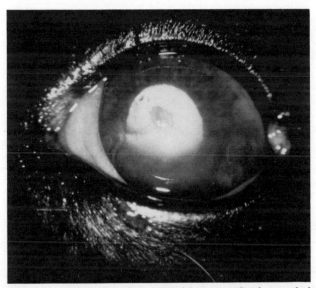

FIGURE 6-7. Viral keratitis characterized by a superficial corneal ulcer that failed to resolve with topical antibiotics. Fluorescent antibody diagnosis for herpesvirus may be diagnostic. Once diagnosed, this ulcer should be treated with topical idoxuridine or trifluridine.

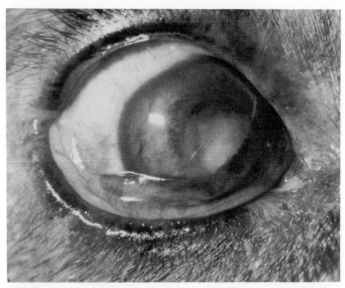

FIGURE 6–8. Fungal keratitis forming a central plaque of infiltrate and fungal hyphae. Scraping of this lesion to obtain material for cytology is usually diagnostic and is of therapeutic value to remove much of the infectious material. Topical natamycin should be applied 3 to 4 times daily for 2 to 3 weeks. Deeper lesions may require a third eyelid or conjunctival flap.

tive keratitis include eyelid coloboma and dermoid. Diagnosis of either of these conditions is usually not difficult; however, for correction through the use of eyelid reconstruction or lamellar keratectomy, they are best referred to a veterinary ophthalmologist.

Corneal sequestrum, a condition unique to the domestic cat, presents with a brown to black, necrotic area within the axial corneal stroma, often surrounded by an area of ulceration and vascularization (Figure 6–9). Resolution requires removal via lamellar keratectomy, best performed by a specialist.

Entropion

Entropion is a rolling in of the eyelid margin and is variable in severity of presentation; one or both lids may be involved. The condition results in contact of the eyelashes with the corneal surface and associated mechanical irritation leading eventually to corneal ulceration. Diagnosis is made upon clinical examination by identification of the eyelid margins and manual retraction by application of digital pressure on the eyelid base. Frequently the

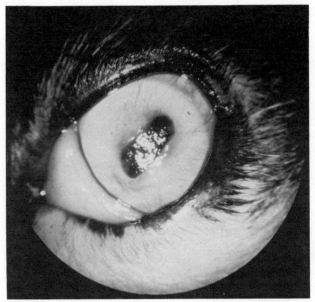

FIGURE 6-9. Corneal sequestrum in a cat characterized by a central black area of necrosis surrounded by corneal granulation. This lesion is best managed by a superficial keratectomy and third eyelid flap.

affected area of lid margin has adherent lacrimal concretions. Secondary signs, including epiphora, blepharospasm, and keratitis, may be present.

Blepharospasm with or without accompanying ulcerative keratitis is often associated with secondary entropion. Following topical anesthesia to relieve the spastic component of the entropion, the true eyelid conformation can be evaluated. Primary hereditary entropion occurs most commonly in the Chow Chow, English Bulldog, and Shar Pei and also in many of the sporting breeds and large working breeds. Senile entropion occurs due to loss of tone of the skin and subcutaneous musculature of the face and usually affects primarily the upper eyelids. Reduction in size of the orbital fat in old or debilitated animals (particularly cats) may lead to enophthalmus and secondary entropion. Eyelid trauma may result in entropion following cicatricial scarring.

If untreated, the corneal pathology accompanying entropion may be progressive, with severe scarring and potential for ulceration and perforation. Animals affected with primary hereditary entropion are usually detected during the first three to six months

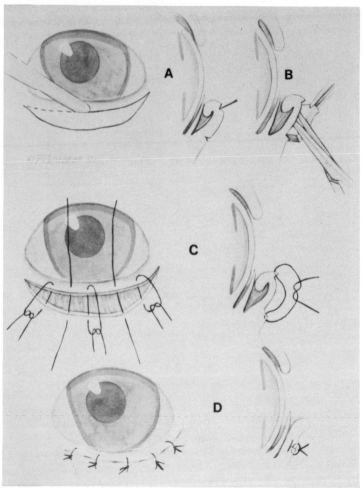

FIGURE 6–10. Hotz-Celsus procedure for entropion correction. The initial incision is made cleanly with a #15 Bard-Parker or #64 Beaver blade held perpendicular to the skin, parallel to and 2 to 4 mm from the lid margin to a depth that includes the orbicularis oculi muscle (*A*). The length of the incision is determined by the length of lid margin involved in the inversion, extending 2 to 3 mm on either side of the inverted portion. The ends of the first incision are joined by a distal elliptical incision, its width previously determined by evaluation of the degree of lid inversion in the unanesthetized animal. If the extent of lid margin inversion is not constant, this incision is adjusted accordingly. Hemorrhage is controlled with digital pressure. The incised area is removed by elevating one end with forceps and excision with scissors (*B*). Three 4-0 silk sutures are placed

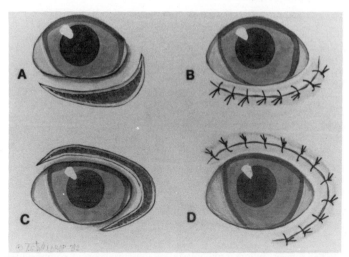

FIGURE 6-11. The Hotz-Celsus procedure may be tailored to each individual case. A sporting breed with lower lid entropion that is more extensive temporally might require different techniques (*A, B*) than the correction (*C, D*) chosen for a patient with entropion with both upper and lower eyelid involvement, commonly seen in the Chow Chow breed. From Peiffer RL Jr et al: Surgery of the canine and feline orbit, adnexa, and globe. Part III: Other structural abnormalities in neoplasia of the eyelids. *Companion Animal Practice* 1:20-36, September 1987.

of life. If the eyelid abnormality is accompanied by corneal ulceration or other significant corneal pathology, immediate surgical correction is indicated. Temporary suturing procedures have been used with some success in very young animals, particularly Shar Peis, where the avoidance of general anesthesia is desirable. Often, however, eventual surgical correction is required in these animals. Surgical excision of an elliptical section of skin approximately 5 mm from the eyelid margin in the area of the entropion is usually curative (Figures 6-10 and 6-11). Meticulous, two-layer closure is necessary for satisfactory cosmetic results. Critical eval-

to divide the incision into quarters (*C*); if the correction appears inadequate immediately following closure, the sutures may be removed and additional tissue removed from the distal edge of the incision. Closure is completed by placing additional sutures approximately 5 mm apart. From Peiffer RL Jr et al: Surgery of the canine and feline orbit, adnexa, and globe. Part III: Other structural abnormalities and neoplasia of the eyelids. *Companion Animal Practice* 1:20-36, September 1987.

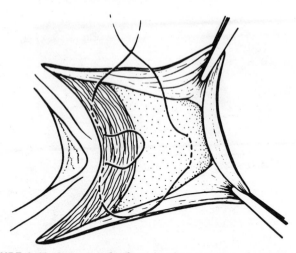

FIGURE 6–12. Suture canthoplasty for the correction of combined entropion and ectropion in the giant breeds. Excision of a lateral canthal cresent-shaped piece of skin is followed by placement of a nonabsorbable 2-0 suture through the orbicularis oculi muscle into the superior and inferior canthal tarsus as depicted. The suture is then carried into the periosteum of the zygomatic arch and tied with adequate tension to restore normal palpebral conformation. From Peiffer RL Jr et al: Surgery of the canine and feline orbit, adnexa, and globe. Part III: Other structural abnormalities and neoplasia of the eyelids. *Companion Animal Practice* 1:20–36, September 1987.

uation of the precise location and degree of the required correction is essential. The giant breeds may present with a combination of entropion and ectropion related to a weakness in the lateral canthal ligament. Surgical correction of multiple eyelid abnormalities may be best performed by a veterinary ophthalmologist; suture canthoplasty (Figure 6–12) provides consistently good results.

Ectopic Cilia

Ectopic cilia should be distinguished from the more common eyelid anomaly, distichiasis. Distichia are supernumerary lashes emanating from the meibomian gland orifice and may contact the cornea and result in epiphora. This condition rarely results in ocular pain or corneal pathology and is discussed more extensively with conditions causing ocular discharge in Chapter 7.

Ectopic cilia are an often elusive source of corneal ulceration. Affected animals are usually less than a year old, and the condition is most often unilateral; although any breed may be affected,

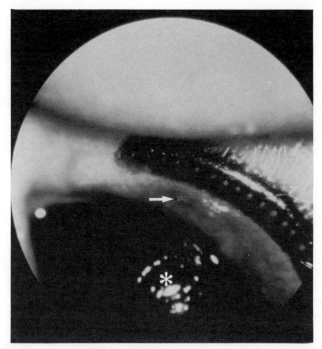

FIGURE 6-13. A highly magnified view of an ectopic cilium (*arrow*) and its associated area of linear, superficial corneal ulceration (∘).

American and English Cocker Spaniels, flat-coated retrievers, and English Bulldogs appear predisposed. These lashes penetrate the palpebral conjunctiva to contact the cornea. The most common location is at the 12 o'clock position, approximately 5 mm from the upper eyelid margin (Figure 6-13). These cilia may be single or multiple and arise from a pigmented or nonpigmented papilla. They are often visible only with the magnification and illumination available with a slitlamp biomicroscope; distichiasis may also be present. Associated ulcers are usually very localized in area and often vertically oriented. Resolution requires microsurgical removal of the offending cilia and its follicle via the palpebral conjunctiva (Figure 6-14).

Neuroparalytic Keratitis

Damage to the facial nerve (VII) results in unilateral facial paralysis and lagophthalmos. The etiology is usually traumatic,

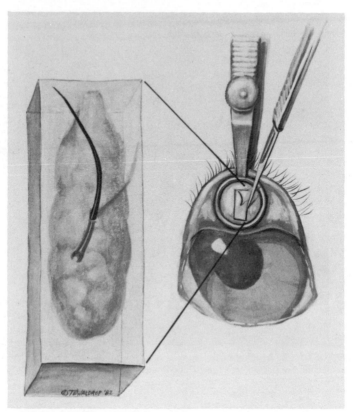

FIGURE 6-14. Tarsoconjunctival resection to manage ectopic cilia. A chalazion forceps is utilized to stabilize the eyelid and control hemorrhage. A #11 Bard-Parker or a #65 Beaver blade is used to excise a rectangle of tarsoconjunctiva containing the ectopic cilia, adjacent meibomian gland, and associated follicle. Occasionally, additional buried cilia and small cystic structures may be encountered in the disection and should be excised as well. Incision is made through the tarsus to a depth of 2 to 3 mm; the excision is completed by elevation with a fine-toothed forceps and undermining dissection with the scalpel or a small scissors. The defect is not sutured; the eyelid margin is left intact. From Peiffer RL Jr et al: Surgery of the canine and feline orbit, adnexa, and globe. Part II: Congenital abnormalities of the eyelid and cilia abnormalities. *Companion Animal Practice* 1:27–38, August 1987.

and drooping of the oral commissure and ear on the affected side are the hallmarks of this condition. Touching the medial canthus does not elicit the normal palpebral reflex. Gentle stimulation of the corneal surface with cotton is associated with backward movement of the head without a blink response. This indicates that the ophthalmic branch of the trigeminal (V) cranial nerve is intact and providing afferent sensation to the cornea, although the motor function to the eyelids is lacking. Such neurologic lagophthalmos is rapidly associated with keratitis related to exposure and drying of the cornea. Immediate therapy involves placement of a temporary tarsorrhaphy to prevent corneal damage (Figure 6–15). A permanent, partial tarsorrhaphy, leaving a small, central palpebral fissure, may be required if the neurological condition does not resolve. Such a procedure would preserve vision in the affected eye but would also require frequent medication to prevent drying of the exposed cornea.

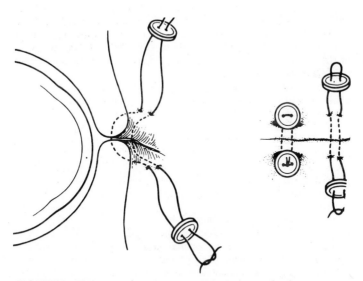

FIGURE 6–15. Suture placement in temporary tarsorrhaphy; cross section and anterior views. Button tension devices are illustrated; IV tubing works equally well. From Peiffer RL Jr et al: Surgery of the canine and feline orbit, adnexa, and globe. Part III: Other structural abnormalities and neoplasia of the eyelids. *Companion Animal Practice* 1:20–36, September 1987.

Neurotrophic Keratitis

Neurological damage to the corneal afferent of the trigeminal nerve results in a lack of corneal sensation although the palpebral motor function remains intact. Absence of corneal sensation may be associated with a reduction in both reflex tear production and blinking. A temporary or permanent canthoplasty to reduce the size of the palpebral fissure is indicated.

GLAUCOMA

Pain associated with acute elevation in intraocular pressure is often overlooked by pet owners. The animals may demonstrate only mild depression and occasionally pain only when the area around the affected eye is touched. Glaucoma is most painful during the acute phase; the slow onset and chronic nature of many cases of glaucoma account for the reduced awareness of this condition by many owners. Blind, enlarged eyes appear to have reduced sensation as a result of the chronically elevated pressure. However, upon removal of an animal's glaucomatous globe, an owner often becomes aware that the animal's attitude has improved, indicating that low-grade pain may indeed be a factor even in chronic cases. Once the eye becomes enlarged to a degree that the animal is unable to completely blink, exposure of the cornea may occur, accompanied by the complications and pain described previously.

Appropriate therapy for glaucoma is dependent upon critical evaluation of the potential for restoration of visual function. Cases of acute glaucoma without globe enlargement usually require surgical management best performed by a veterinary ophthalmologist. Chronically enlarged eyes carry a poor visual prognosis with therapy directed at resolution of discomfort and providing a cosmetic result. Options include: enucleation, cyclocryosurgery, implantation of an intraocular prosthesis, and injection of gentamicin to cause pharmacologic ablation of the ciliary body. Of these procedures, enucleation is the most predictable, although the cosmetic result is not satisfactory to some pet owners. The result may be improved somewhat by placement of a 22-mm methylmethacrylate sphere in the orbital space to reduce the sunken appearance of the orbit postoperatively. Removal of the globe should be performed with care to leave the extraocular tissues to be sutured around the sphere and fix it in place within the orbit. Enucleation with histopathologic evaluation is the procedure of choice if intraocular neoplasia is suspected.

Intravitreal injection of gentamicin (25 mg combined with 1 mg dexamethasone; an equal volume of vitreous is first aspirated) is usually successful in reducing the intraocular pressure and may be performed without general anesthesia; however, the postoperative results are less predictable than the other options. Cataract and intraocular hemorrhage are frequent sequellae.

Implantation of an intraocular prosthesis requires some specialized instrumentation and careful surgical technique to avoid damage to the corneal endothelium with resultant postoperative corneal opacification.

Cyclocryosurgery offers somewhat less predictable results, with more than one procedure occasionally required. Postoperative chemosis and discomfort are most pronounced with this procedure.

UVEITIS

Intraocular inflammation, regardless of cause, is often accompanied by pain. Epiphora and blepharospasm may be present, particularly in bright light.

7 | Ocular Discharge

Simon M. Petersen-Jones
and Robert L. Peiffer, Jr.

In this chapter we consider ophthalmic disorders in which serous, mucoid, or purulent ocular discharge is the most prominent sign. Conditions are discussed under the heading that describes the discharge with which they most commonly present; however, certain conditions can present with differing discharge types.

INTRODUCTION

Discharge from the eye typically occurs as either an inflammatory exudation from the adnexa (eyelids, conjunctiva, nasolacrimal system); excessive reflex tearing in response to corneal and/or conjunctival irritation; or obstruction of the nasolacrimal excretory system, with resultant tear overflow. Less commonly ocular discharge results from an orbital abscess draining via a tract to the conjunctival surface. Compromise of the ocular tunic may allow the leakage of intraocular fluids and, if infection is involved, purulent exudate.

Patients with ocular discharge can be readily segregated into two groups, those with and those without obvious external ocular disease. The signs of inflammation of the adnexa are the same as those of other tissues of the body: vascular dilation, tissue edema, and exudation. Ulcerative or nonulcerative keratitis is usually accompanied by discharge. Serous or mucoid discharge may accompany primary intraocular disease, such as uveitis or glaucoma; however, as it is not usually the most prominent presenting sign, these conditions are considered elsewhere.

Ocular discharge can be classified by its consistency and components (serous, mucoid, or purulent), its duration, and/or its association with other ocular signs. Serous discharge may be associated with ocular irritation resulting from such factors as distichiasis or a hairy caruncle. Signs of mild ocular pain and in some cases corneal pathology may also be present in such cases. Inadequate tear drainage results in a serous discharge but with no signs of ocular pain or discomfort. Tenacious mucopurulent exudation is the hallmark of keratoconjunctivitis sicca (KCS). Purulent discharge is usually indicative of an infectious process.

Clinical history can be helpful in reaching a diagnosis. For example, patients with KCS usually have a long history of ocular discharge that has responded transiently to topical medication. Serous discharge associated with congenital abnormalities of the nasolacrimal excretory system typically is not notable until 6 to 12 months of age, although the underlying problem has been present since birth. Conjunctivitis may have a history of being an acute or chronic problem, depending on its etiology.

A few simple diagnostic tools are required for the diagnosis and monitoring of patients with ocular discharge. A Schirmer tear test should be used to check the tear production of all patients with external ocular disease, particularly those with a history of chronic ocular discharge. Rose bengal stain in a sensitive indicator of epithelial well-being. Exfoliative conjunctival cytology is useful in the investigation of conjunctivitis. The ocular surface should be cultured if the problem is chronic or has failed to respond to medication. The nasolacrimal system can be evaluated by observing the drainage of fluorescein added to the conjunctival sac and by punctal cannulation and irrigation.

SEROUS DISCHARGE

The inability of the nasolacrimal system to drain the volume of tears produced by the patient results in a serous discharge due to tear overflow (*epiphora*). Both impaired tear drainage and increased tear production due to ocular irritation can result in epiphora.

Increased Tear Production

Tear production is reflexly increased by ocular irritation or pain. In patients with distichiasis, ectopic cilia, trichiasis, or entropion, the cornea is irritated by cilia, resulting in increased tear production and tear overflow.

Distichiasis is common in dogs and rare in cats. The abnormally positioned cilia emerge from the eyelid margin, and, if thick and inflexible, they may penetrate the precorneal tear film and abrade the cornea. Most cases are asymptomatic and need not be treated. Clinical signs of pain and/or corneal lesions are indications for permanent destruction or removal of the follicles of the offending cilia. The follicles are positioned in or adjacent to the meibomian glands. Various procedures have been used in the treatment of distichiasis, including electroepilation, cryosurgery, and lid-splitting procedures. In our experience careful surgical excision (Figures 7-1 and 7-2) produces the most consistent results, with infrequent complications such as regrowth and lid scarring.

Aberrant cilia within the eyelid may also emerge through the palpebral conjunctiva and are then known as ectopic cilia. Their most common position is midway along the upper eyelid. At this site they abrade the cornea with each movement of the upper eyelid and may cause a corresponding vertical band of keratitis or superficial corneal ulceration. Treatment consists of destruction or surgical removal of the offending hair follicle (see Chapter 6 on ocular pain).

The misdirection of facial hair onto the cornea is known as *trichiasis*. Upper eyelid agenesis in cats, prominent nasal folds in brachycephalic breeds of dogs, and previous eyelid trauma (including poorly performed lid-splitting procedures) can all result in trichiasis. Trichiasis may cause a superficial keratitis; for example, nasal fold trichiasis of brachycephalic dogs often induces a medial pigmentary keratitis. When trichiasis does result in clinical problems, the offending hairs should be removed or redirected with a modified entropion procedure.

Hairs commonly grow from the caruncle of certain breeds of dog, notably the Lhasa Apso (Figure 7-3). In some individuals these hairs cause slight ocular irritation, with epiphora frequently the primary complaint. Such cases are best managed by medial canthoplasty.

Entropion results in corneal irritation by the hairs of the turned-in eyelid. Surgical eversion of the eyelid corrects the deformity and relieves the irritation.

Impaired Tear Drainage

Tear drainage is a complex process. In the dog and cat, the precorneal tear film enters the nasolacrimal drainage system via the two puncta positioned on the upper and lower eyelid margins at the medial canthal region. The majority of drainage occurs via the lower punctum. Blinking results in tears being squeezed into the canaliculi, which themselves have a pumping action and valve mechanism. Gravity may also aid tear drainage.

The overall tear-drainage process may be assessed by the addition of fluorescein dye to the precorneal tear film. In the individual with a functional drainage system, the dye appears at the corresponding nostril a few minutes after administration. In some brachycephalic breeds, drainage to the nasopharynx may occur. The physical patency of the nasolacrimal system itself may be assessed by punctal cannulation and irrigation. This procedure does not assess the physiological drainage process; the nasolacrimal sys-

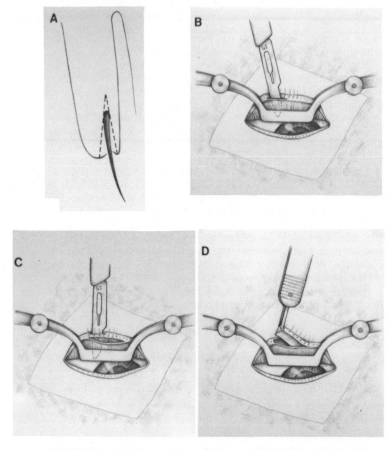

FIGURE 7-1. Partial tarsal plate excision for distichiasis: *A,* Cross-section of distichia-bearing eyelid. Dashed line shows incision required for partial tarsal place excision. *B,* Bedford distichiasis clamp is placed on eyelid. With a #15 scalpel blade, an incision is made to the required depth from the eyelid margin on the conjunctival side of the distichia. *C,* A second incision parallel to the first is made from the eyelid margin on the skin side of the distichia. This results in a wedge-shaped piece of eyelid tissue including the part of the tarsal plate bearing the follicles of the distichia. *D,* The distichia-bearing wedge of eyelid tissue is then excised.

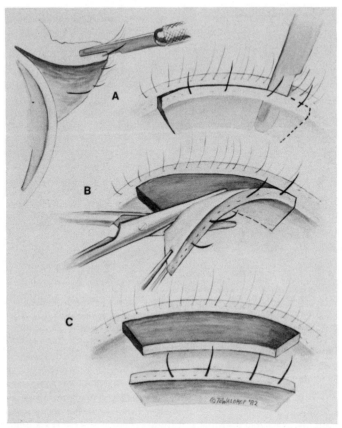

FIGURE 7–2. An alternative technique for distichiasis is tarsoconjunctival resection: A, The lid is held with tissue forceps or stabilized in a chalazion clamp. The ends of the cilia-bearing tarsoconjunctival strip to be excised are demarcated by incising through the palpebral conjunctiva at the lid margin perpendicular to the margin to a depth of 2 mm (deep enough to reach the tarsus and include the distichia). This incision should be approximately 5 mm long. B, A #15 Bard-Parker or #64 Beaver blade is used to split the lid perpendicular to the lid margin to the length and depth established by the initial incision; the lid is split at or slightly bulbar to the level of the meibomian gland orifices, as necessary, to include the distichia. C, The base of the cilia-bearing strip is excised with small scissors. Hemorrhage is controlled with direct pressure. The cutaneous portion of the lid margin is left intact. From Peiffer RL Jr et al: Surgery of the canine and feline orbit, adnexa, and globe. Part II: Congenital abnormalities of the eyelid and cilia abnormalities. *Companion Animal Practice* 1:27–38, August 1987.

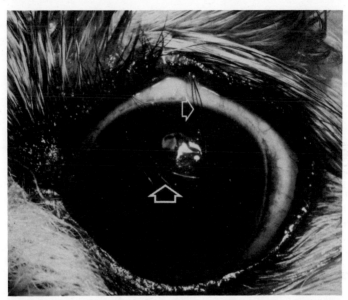

FIGURE 7-3. Trichiasis related to a hairy caruncle and distichiasis in a Lhasa Apso. The hairs from the medial canthus are floating across the surface of the cornea in the tear film (*arrow*); the distichiasis (*small arrow*) is an example of districhiasis with several hairs emerging from a single follicle.

tem may be physically patent, yet epiphora still occurs. This condition is common in some breeds, notably Toy and Miniature Poodles and Persian cats. The shallow medial canthal lake and/or mild lower medial entropion of these breeds results in tears being squeezed onto the face rather than into the nasolacrimal system. Surgical eversion of the medial lower lid may prove beneficial in such cases (Figure 7-4).

Agenesis of the lower punctum is a relatively common cause of epiphora. The lower canaliculis is usually present, and only the punctal opening is absent. Occasionally a cystic swelling may be present (Figure 7-5). Cannulation and irrigation of the upper punctum cause a slight bulging of the lower canaliculis, thus indicating where the surgeon must incise to create a lower punctal opening (Figure 7-6). Micropunctum is another abnormality that may be readily treated surgically. The *three-snips* procedure is used to enlarge such a punctum. This is carried out by the insertion of one blade of a fine pair of straight iris scissors into the punctum. Two parallel cuts produce a small flap of conjunctiva overlying the canaliculis; this is then excised (the third snip) to leave an

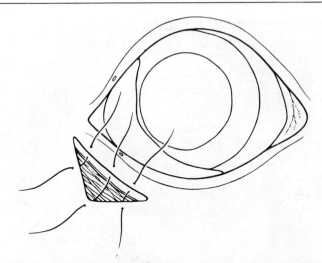

FIGURE 7–4. A triangular wedge of skin and orbicularis oculi muscle is excised to manage lower eyelid entropion with associated epiphora in Toy and Miniature Poodles and Persian cats. The apex of the triangle should be opposite the lower puncta, and incision depth should be conservative to avoid trauma to the lower canaliculus. Closure is with 4-0 silk. From Peiffer RL JR et al: Surgery of the canine and feline orbit, adnexa, and globe. Part III: Other structural abnormalities and neoplasia of the eyelids. *Companion Animal Practice* 1:20–36, September 1987.

enlarged opening into the canaliculis. More extensive agenesis of the nasolacrimal duct system does occur (fortunately, rarely) and may be more difficult to correct.

Acquired blockage of the nasolacrimal system may result from lid trauma or surgery to the canalicular region. Scarring following severe conjunctivitis may occlude the system. Such scarring may result from feline viral rhinotracheitis–induced conjunctivitis in younger cats. Neoplasia may also occlude the drainage system. Examples include eyelid neoplasia in the canalicular region and compression of the nasolacrimal duct by tumors such as maxillary sinus carcinomas; radiographs of the skull are indicated in older patients with acquired epiphora in the absence of other causes.

MUCOID DISCHARGE

Mucus is an important constituent of the precorneal tear film. Its normal fate is to be squeezed out onto the skin at the medial canthal area, where it dries and drops off or is wiped away. Dogs

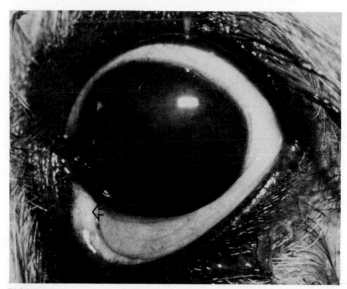

FIGURE 7-5. Congenital absence of the lower punctum in a 5-year-old Lhasa Apso presented with epiphora; in this case, a cyst is present at the area of the occluded canaliculus (*arrow*).

such as Dobermans and Weimeraners, which have a degree of enophthalmia, often accumulate mucus in the deep medial lacrimal lake. The mucus is not indicative of ocular pathology.

Increased mucus production may accompany increased lacrimation early in the course of conjunctivitis. Patients with allergic, viral, and chlamydial conjunctivitis may present with a mucoserous discharge. Signs of inflammation and ocular irritation will also be present. If secondary bacterial infections occur, the discharge will become mucopurulent.

A conjunctival scraping taken early in the course of a conjunctivitis can be useful in establishing a diagnosis. A surface scraping of cells may be taken using a Kimura spatula or the blunt end of a #15 scalpel blade. The collected bead of material is gently smeared onto a clean microscope slide, air dried, and alcohol fixed. Gram staining and Giemsa staining are usually performed. Commercial "quick stains," which produce an acceptably stained slide ready to be examined a few minutes after performing the scrape, may be used.

The normal conjunctival scrape reveals sheets of epithelial cells, mucus, and the occasional inflammatory cell such as neutrophils and lymphocytes. In man a scraping from a case of allergic con-

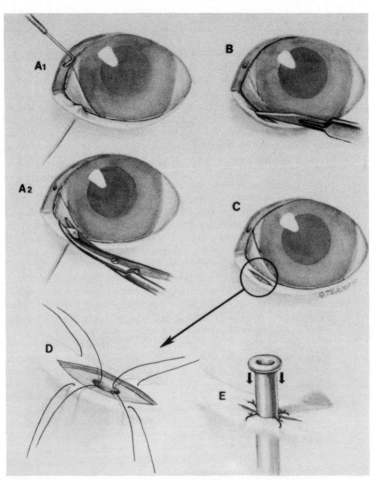

FIGURE 7-6. Punctoplasty for punctal hypoplasia or aplasia. *A*, The location of the lower puncta is identified by irrigation from the upper puncta (if present) or by retrograde cannulation from the nasal mucosa; the conjunctiva overlying the canaliculi may be snipped with a pair of scissors if no lower puncta is present. *B*, Enlargement of a hypoplastic puncta is most readily performed by inserting a #11 Bard-Parker or #65 Beaver blade into the puncta and creating a slit to enlarge the opening or by using the three-snip technique described in the text. To ensure patency during healing (*C*), the mucosa of the canaliculus may be sutured to the conjunctiva with 7-0 absorbable suture (*D*), and/or silastic tubing with a flanged end may be inserted down the nasolacrimal duct and fixed at the nasal orifice (*E*). These alternatives are seldom required, and the majority of cases will heal nicely without suturing or cannulation. From Peiffer RL Jr et al: Surgery of the canine and feline orbit, adnexa, and globe. Part IV: The nasolacrimal system. *Companion Animal Practice* 1:5–11, October 1987.

junctivitis usually contains a few eosinophils; this may also be true of allergic conjunctivitis in animals. The allergic reaction, however, may be due to a bacterial toxin (e.g., staphylococcal toxins) and not the primary cause of the conjunctivitis itself. Initially, conjunctival scrapings from cases of viral conjunctivitis show a preponderance of mononuclear cells. As secondary bacterial infections develop, neutrophils become more common. Scrapings from cats with chlamydial conjunctivitis usually reveal a mixed neutrophil and mononuclear response. The presence of chlamydial inclusion bodies within the cytoplasm of epithelial cells confirms the diagnosis, but they are not commonly found.

Fluorescent antibody techniques are available for the identification of chlamydial and viral antigens in conjunctival scrapes. These are particularly useful for the diagnosis of feline viral rhinotracheitis and feline chlamydial conjunctivitis. The inflammatory cell picture of long-standing cases of conjunctivitis usually shows a mixed cellular response and is therefore less of a diagnostic guide than scrapes taken early in the course of the disease. Gram staining of scrapes can give a rapid indication of bacterial involvement and helps in the selection of an appropriate antibiotic. Bacterial isolation and sensitivity testing can later confirm that the appropriate antibiotic was selected.

Foreign bodies within the conjunctival sac may induce an increased mucus production in addition to a reflex increase in tear production. Signs of conjunctival inflammation and irritation will also be present. The possibility of the presence of conjunctival foreign bodies makes a complete examination of the conjunctival sac mandatory when conjunctival inflammation is present. The use of a topical anesthetic is especially useful when examining the bulbar surface of the third eyelid.

PURULENT DISCHARGE

Purulent or mucopurulent discharge can be a feature of a number of conditions. Bacterial conjunctivitis (primary or secondary) results in a purulent ocular discharge; in some cases, there may also be a concurrent blepharitis or keratitis. The bacteria involved are often those found as normal skin flora. When the host's resistance is lowered, or something damages surface epithelial cells, certain bacteria may become established and result in an infection. Bacteria, including those considered as "potential pathogens," may be cultured in low numbers from the conjunctival sac of over 50 percent of normal dogs. The bacteria involved probably represent transient contaminants from the skin rather than a stable flora.

A chronic mucopurulent discharge with little or no conjunctival or corneal pathology is typical of a chronic dacryocystitis. Digital pressure over the lacrimal sac region results in expression of pus from the nasolacrimal puncta. Dacryocystitis is often due to the presence of a nasolacrimal foreign body. Gentle irrigation from upper to lower puncta and vice versa will expel pus, some of which should be collected for bacteriology. Irrigation may help express any foreign bodies from the lacrimal sac. Care must be taken not to force-flush a foreign body into the portion of na-solacrimal duct surrounded by bone. At such a site removal is much more difficult. The introduction of a radio-opaque fluid into the nasolacrimal duct followed by radiography (dacryocys-tography) may be of use in identifying the site of the nasolacrimal obstructions, as may threading a monofilament thread down the nasolacrimal duct. A chronic dacryocystitis may be refractory to treatment and require daily lavage of the nasolacrimal system in order to achieve a cure. Antibiotic solutions may be used for such lavage.

Foreign bodies that have penetrated through the conjunctiva into the periocular tissues may result in abscess formation, sinus formation, and the discharge of purulent material into the con-junctival sac. Retrobulbar abscesses may also, on occasion, dis-charge pus into the conjunctival sac. Sinuses emptying into the conjunctival sac sometimes have their origin at a surprising dis-tance from the eye. Foreign bodies within the wall of the com-mon pharynx or nasopharynx may result in abscesses that even-tually discharge via the conjunctival sac. Such abscesses should be drained and thoroughly searched for foreign bodies, and the appropriate antibiotics should be prescribed.

A chronic, tenacious mucopurulent ocular discharge that re-sponds transiently to any topical treatment is typical of kerato-conjunctivitis sicca (KCS). The discharge accumulates within the conjunctival fornices and is often adherent to the cornea. Con-junctival and corneal changes rapidly develop. Secondary bacte-rial infection is common, with a heavy growth of bacteria being isolated from the conjunctival sac of many patients with KCS. Rapid-onset KCS may result in serious corneal ulceration, and such cases are ocular emergencies. More slowly developing KCS usually results in a chronic nonulcerative superficial keratitis. The amount of corneal pathology varies among individual cases and does not necessarily follow the level of tear production as mea-sured by the Schirmer tear test (STT). STT readings below 10 mm/minute are suggestive of KCS. Cats less commonly develop KCS than dogs. When felines do develop KCS, corneal pigmenta-tion and scarring do not usually occur to the same extent as they do in dogs.

Congenital aplasia or hypoplasia of the tear-producing glands may result in congenital KCS. Prior excision of the gland of the

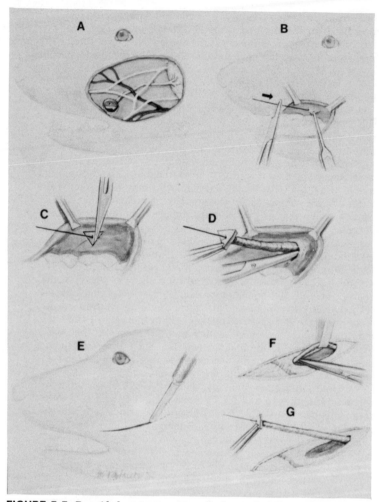

FIGURE 7-7. Parotid duct transposition: *A,* Surgical anatomy. Note that the parotid duct lies deep to the facial vein and the buccal nerves on the surface of the masseter muscle. *B,* The parotid duct is cannulated with 0 or 00 nylon monofilament suture, the tip of which has been previously flamed smooth. The orifice of the duct lies just above the carnassial tooth and should not be confused with that of the zygomatic gland, which is just above the molar and usually more dorsal. The cannula is inserted while the adjacent buccal mucosa is grasped with fine-toothed forceps and anterior traction is applied to straighten the duct. Magnification will facilitate this procedure as well as the surgery. When in place, the cannula may be palpated through the skin and its position positively identified.

third eyelid predisposes to KCS. Damage to the tear-producing glands due to canine distemper adenitis or by the toxic side effects of certain drugs, such as phenazopyridine (in dogs only) or sulfadiazine, can result in KCS. Denervation of the parasympathetic supply to the lacrimal and third eyelid glands causes KCS; in such neurogenic cases, nasal secretions of the ipsilateral side are usually also reduced, resulting in a dry nostril. Trauma to the gland and/or its innervation is also a recognized cause of dry eye. The majority of cases of KCS are idiopathic. Genetic tendencies to KCS exist in certain breeds of dog, notably the Lhasa Apso and the West Highland White Terrier.

KCS is treated by twice daily copious irrigation of the eye with sterile saline and regular administration of artificial tears. Antibiotics are indicated when secondary bacterial infections develop. If the cornea is not ulcerated, topical corticosteroids used with care may help reduce the extent of corneal scarring and relieve some of the discomfort and irritation. If corneal ulceration develops, a third eyelid or conjunctival flap may be necessary to save the eye and aid healing. Oral pilocarpine (at a dose rate of 1 to 4 drops of a 1% solution twice daily) acts as a lacrimogenic and may be of benefit if some functional glandular tissue remains; pilocarpine is especially effective in treating neurogenic cases of KCS. The successful medical management of KCS demands significant client education and participation. Success of treatment depends on the severity of the disease and on the ability of the owner to medicate the animal regularly. The ocular contact time of tear substitutes is short, and they should ideally be applied hourly for optimal benefit. Artificial tear ointments have a longer ocular contact time than drops. The STT levels should be regularly monitored during treatment.

Topical cyclosporine, a T-cell immunosuppressive agent, has recently been shown to be beneficial in the medical management of KCS; twice daily application of a 2.0% solution will re-

---

C, The peripapillary oral mucosa is incised with a liberal border about the duct orifice, taking care not to damage the duct. A triangular mucosal incision is shown; a 5 or 6 mm dermal biopsy punch may also be used.

D, Working directly through the oral incision and using the tips of fine scissors to spread and bluntly dissect, the duct is isolated for about 1–2 cm. *E*, A 3–4 cm facial incision is made along the course of the duct; the duct is isolated and freed by blunt dissection. *F*, The duct is not handled directly but elevated and retracted with umbilical tape. *G*, The duct and its papilla are gently pulled into the facial incision. The duct must not be kinked, twisted, or handled traumatically during this procedure. From Peiffer RL Jr et al: Surgery of the canine and feline orbit, adnexa, and globe. Part IV: The nasolacrimal system. *Companion Animal Practice* 1:5–11, October 1987.

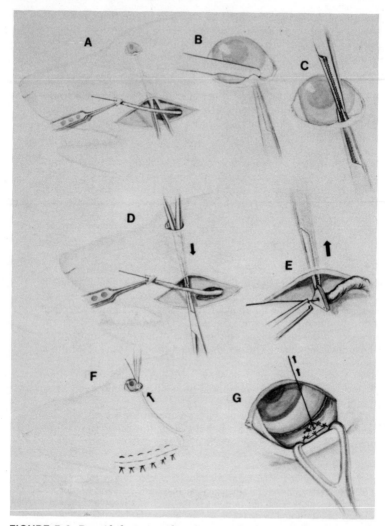

FIGURE 7-8. Parotid duct transplant (continued). *A,* A tunnel is made with straight mosquito forceps from the facial incision to the inferior temporal conjunctival sac. *B,* The conjunctiva is incised to allow the tip of the forceps to be completely free. *C–D,* The tunneled forceps is used to pull a second pair of mosquito forceps into the tunnel and down to the facial incision.

E, The second forceps is used to grasp the mucosa adjacent to the papilla and pull it up to the eye. Care should be taken at this time to be sure the duct is not stretched, kinked, or twisted.

sult in increases in Schirmer tear test values with regression of clinical signs in a significant percentage of KCS patients. We recommend its usage in conjunction with irrigation, artificial tears, and antibiotic-corticosteroid combinations; as with other medical approaches to KCS, lifelong administration is required.

If the STT levels remain low and medical treatment fails to halt the progression of corneal pathology, parotid duct transposition (PDT) should be considered (Figures 7-7 and 7-8). In most cases the PDT works well to control the disease. Progression of corneal pathology is usually halted and often reversed to some extent. Salivary epiphora may be a problem in some cases, and blepharitis can result. Crystallization of salivary salts onto the cornea and eyelashes may also cause irritation. Continued use of occasional lubricants and topical antibiotics and corticosteroids, as well as daily irrigation, will minimize these problems. Despite the possible complications, PDT has saved the eyesight and relieved the ocular discomfort associated with KCS of many of our patients.

F and *G*, Using 5 to 7 sutures of 6-0 or 7-0 absorbable suture, the peripapillary mucosa is apposed to the conjunctiva of the inferior cul-de-sac. A lateral canthotomy may be used to enhance exposure in small dogs with tight eyelids but is usually not necessary. The skin incision is closed in two layers, and the buccal mucosa is closed with a single absorbable mattress suture. From Peiffer RL Jr et al: Surgery of the canine and feline orbit, adnexa, and globe. Part IV: The nasolacrimal system. *Companion Animal Practice* 1:5–11, October 1987.

Suggested Readings

Aguirre, G.: Symposium on Ophthalmology. Vet. Clin. North Am. 3, September, 1973.

Bistner, S.I., Aguirre, G., and Batik, G.: Atlas of Veterinary Ophthalmic Surgery, W.B. Saunders Company, Philadelphia, 1977.

Blogg, J.R.: The Eye in Veterinary Practice. Extraocular Disease, W.B. Saunders Company, Philadelphia, 1980.

Gelatt, K.N.: Veterinary Ophthalmology. Lea and Febiger, Philadelphia, 1981.

Magrane, W.G.: Canine Ophthalmology. Lea and Febiger, Philadelphia, 1977.

Peiffer, R.L. (ed.): Comparative Ophthalmic Pathology. C.C Thomas, Springfield, Ill., 1983.

Peiffer, R.L. (ed.): Symposium on Ophthalmology. Vet. Clin. North Am. 10(2) May, 1980.

Rubin, L.F.: Atlas of Veterinary Ophthalmoscopy. Lea and Febiger, Philadelphia, 1974.

Saunders, L.A. and Rubin, L.F.: Ophthalmic Pathology of Animals. S. Karger, Basel, 1975.

Slatter, D.H.: Fundamentals of Veterinary Ophthalmology. W.B. Saunders Company, Philadelphia, 1981.

Index

Note: Numbers in *italic* indicate illustrations; numbers followed by the letter t indicate tables.